Cardiac MRI Certification Exam

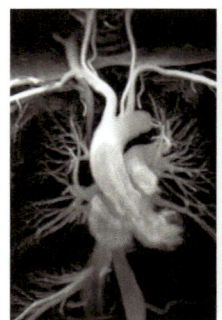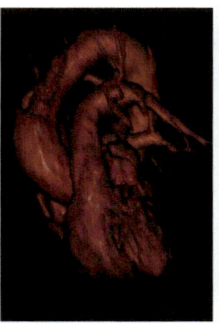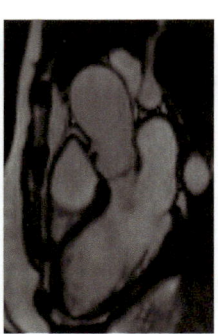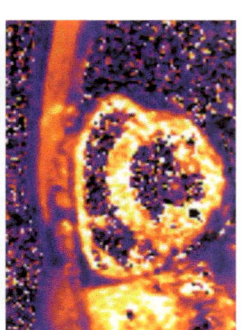

Sadeer G. Al-Kindi • Scott E. Janus

Cardiac MRI Certification Exam

150 Questions and Review

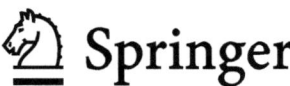

Springer

Sadeer G. Al-Kindi
University Hospitals Cleveland
Medical Center
Cleveland, OH, USA

Scott E. Janus
University Hospitals Cleveland
Medical Center
Cleveland, OH, USA

ISBN 978-3-031-25965-4   ISBN 978-3-031-25966-1   (eBook)
https://doi.org/10.1007/978-3-031-25966-1

This Springer imprint is published by the registered company Springer Nature Switzerland AG
The registered company address is: Gewerbestrasse 11, 6330 Cham, Switzerland

Preface

Cardiovascular magnetic resonance imaging (CMR) is now an essential part of cardiology training. These 150 questions and reviews provide a comprehensive and easily readable education tool for trainees and cardiologists in preparing for the CMR Certification Examinations. This review contains 150 multiple-choice questions similar to topics found on the board examination and are supported by concise summaries and explanations with links to up-to-date resources and literature. The questions explore a wide breadth of cardiac pathologies from ischemic to valvular to congenital heart disease.

Drs. Al-Kindi and Janus are both certified by American Board of Internal Medicine© in Internal Medicine and Cardiovascular Medicine, certified by National Board of Echocardiography©, and in Cardiac Magnetic Resonance Imaging by Certification Board of Cardiovascular Magnetic Resonance (CBCMR) ©. We would like to thank our co-authors/co-contributors Dr. Imran Rashid and Dr. Sanjay Rajagopalan for their partial review of the materials. We must thank our wonderful nurses (Sara Palker and Ellen Musarra), technologists (Jason Eastman, Bridget Razem, June James, and Amanda Maguire), and administrative personnel (Daniela Riggio) for helping take care of our patients and acquire these images. We would like to thank Drs. Hajjari, Chami, Mously, Karnib, Chahine, Al Jammal, and Badhwar for their help with reviewing the cases. We additionally need to thank our patients for the images and teachings they have provided, and lastly our families for the support along this journey.

Cleveland, OH   Sadeer G. Al-Kindi
Cleveland, OH   Scott E. Janus

Contents

Chapter 1
Basics of MRI

1. Match the correct series with the correct repetition time (TR) and time to echo (TE).

(A) T1 (Long/Long) and T2 (Short/Short)
(B) T1 (Short/Short) and T2 (Long/Long)
(C) T1 (Long/Short) and T2 (Short/Long)
(D) T1 (Short/Long) and T2 (Long/Short)

The correct answer is B. On spin echo imaging, the repetition time (TR) and the echo time (TE) are used to help weigh the image and control image contrast. To produced T1-weighted image, a short TE and TR is required. T2-Weighted images require long TR and long TE as shown in figure [1].

S. G. Al-Kindi, S. E. Janus, *Cardiac MRI Certification Exam*, https://doi.org/10.1007/978-3-031-25966-1_1

T1-Weighted (Short TR/Short TE)

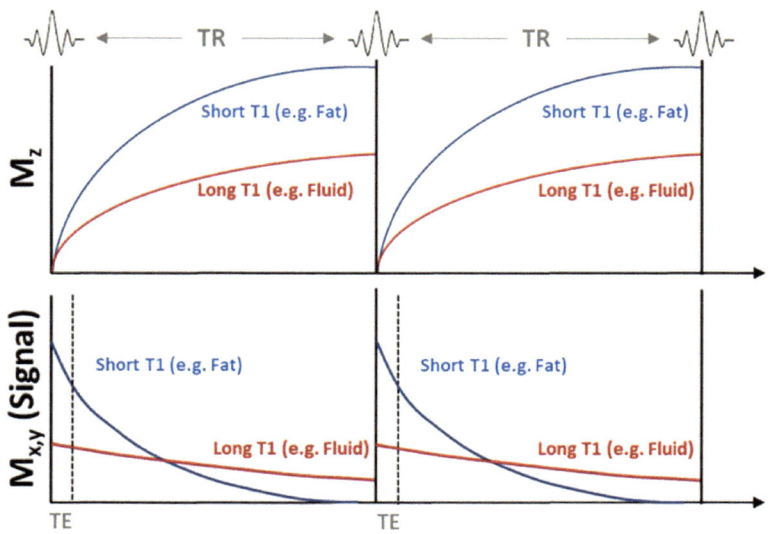

T2-Weighted (Long TR/Long TE)

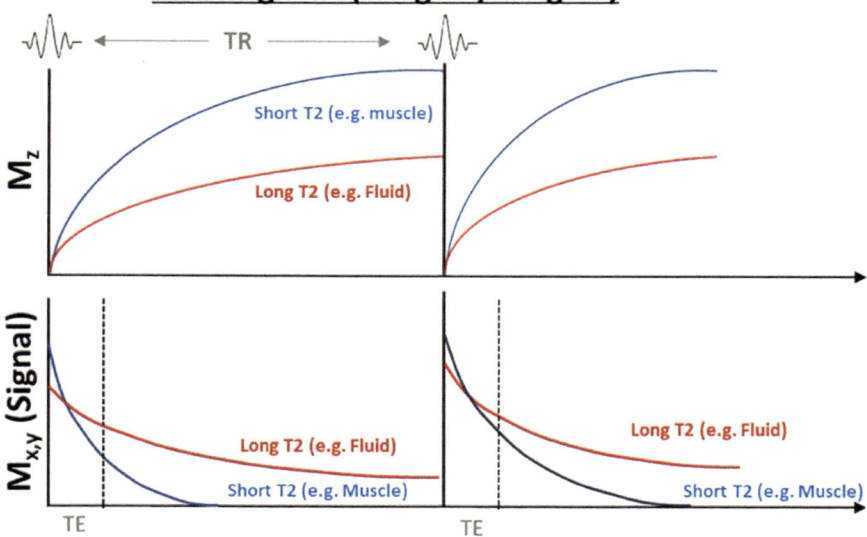

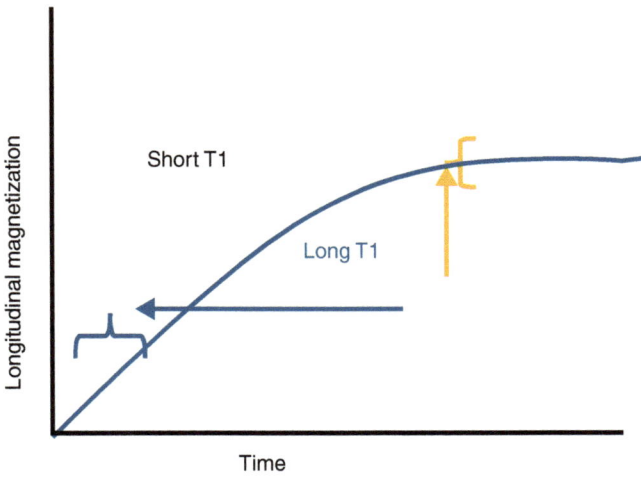

Blue arrow demonstrates larger
differentiation of tissues based on T1
compared to yellow arrow

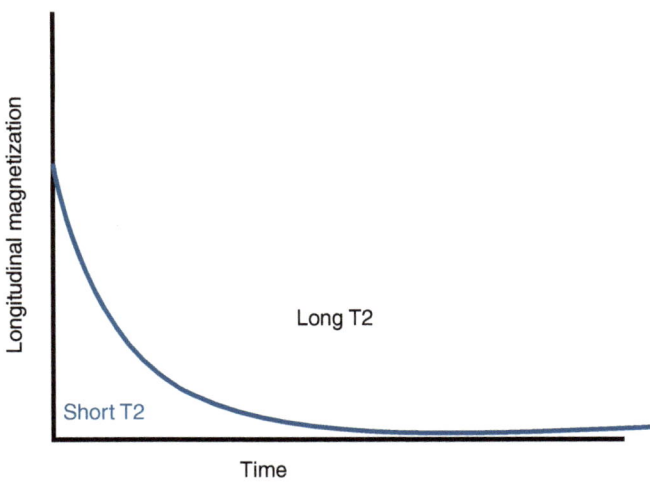

2. How would you describe this patient's LV mass and size indexed for a male?

Measurements

Volumetric Analysis

		LV
EDV	[ml]	309
	[ml/m²]	165
ESV	[ml]	236
	[ml/m²]	126
CO	[L/min]	4.46
	[L/min/m²]	2.39
MASS	[g]	145
	[g/m²]	78

(A) Dilated left ventricle size with increased mass
(B) Dilated left ventricle size with normal mass
(C) Normal left ventricle size with normal mass
(D) Normal left ventricle size with increased mass

The correct answer is B. The normal range for LVEDV/BSA is 50–108/m² and LV Mass 39–85 g/m² [2].

	Male			Female		
	Average	Lower limit	Upper limit	Average	Lower limit	Upper limit
EF (%)	64	49	79	66	52	79
Mass (g)	121	66	176	83	41	125
Mass/BSA (g/m²)	62	39	85	49	30	68
EDV (ml)	155	95	215	123	78	167
EDV/BSA (ml/m²)	79	50	108	73	50	96
ESV (ml)	55	28	85	43	21	64
ESV/BSA (ml/m²)	29	11	47	25	10	40
SV (ml)	103	61	83	83	52	114
SV/BSA (ml/m²)	52	33	72	49	33	64

Kawel-Boehm et al. [2]

3. The magnetohydrodynamic effect will cause:

(A) Difficulties with gating secondary to changes in the EKG leads
(B) Overestimation of aortic valve gradients
(C) Disrupt the compressible fluid dynamics
(D) Cause significant burns to the patient if persistent

The correct answer is A. The magnetohydrodynamic effect is a physical phenomenon describing motion of conducting fluid under influence of magnet, and can increase the amplitude of T wave thus hindering correct R peak detection [3]. The magnetohydrodynamic effect does not change the estimation of aortic valve gradients, as this is related to velocity encoding [4]. The magnetohydrodynamic effect does not alter the fluid dynamics and certainly does not cause physical burns to the patient.

4. India ink artifact can be corrected by:

(A) Changing the echo time due to interaction of chemical shifts at the fat–water interface
(B) Changing the velocity encoding
(C) Changing phase and frequency encoding directions
(D) Parallel imaging

The correct answer is A. The black boundary artifact also known as the Indian ink artifact is the result of artificially created black lines at the fat–water interface. It results in sharp delineation leading to the imagination of someone outlining these interfaces with wet ink. These artifacts can be reduced by changing to a spin echo sequence, changing the echo time, increasing the bandwidth, or using fat suppression [5]. Velocity encoding is for the determination of gradient [4]. Changing phase and frequency encoding would not solve the problem due to still having the chemical shift and the incorrect echo time. Parallel imaging decreases the time for imaging [6], but would not affect the chemical shift.

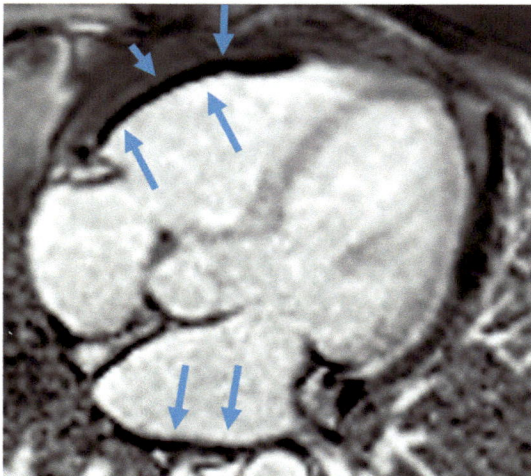

Blue arrows demonstrate Indian Ink Artifact caused by chemical shift at fat water interface

5. The maximum specific absorption rate (SAR) for the body for "normal" level MRI is:

(A) 4 W/kg
(B) 3 W/kg
(C) 2 W/kg
(D) 1 W/kg

The correct answer is C. The maximum specific absorption rate (SAR) for the whole body is 2.0 W/kg [7]. According to the same document, the maximum temperature limit is 39 degree Celsius or 1 degree increase. Head is allowed 3.0 W/kg. First level body is allowed up to 4.0 W/kg [8].

6. What is the normal myocardial value on T1 relaxation time imaging on 1.5 Tesla?

(A) 500–700 msec
(B) 700–900 msec
(C) 900–1100 msec
(D) 1100–1300 msec

The correct answer is C. On a 1.5-Tesla scanner, the typical value of normal myocardium is around 900–1100 msec, but this is highly dependent on the sequence used (MOLLI, shMOLLI, etc) [9]. On a 3.0-Tesla, the normal myocardial valve is between 1100 and 1200 msec [10]. Answer choices A–B is seen with severe fatty infiltration or iron deposition which shortens the T1 values [11]. Answer choice D is seen in amyloid infiltration, fibrosis of inflammation where the T1 values are elevated [9].

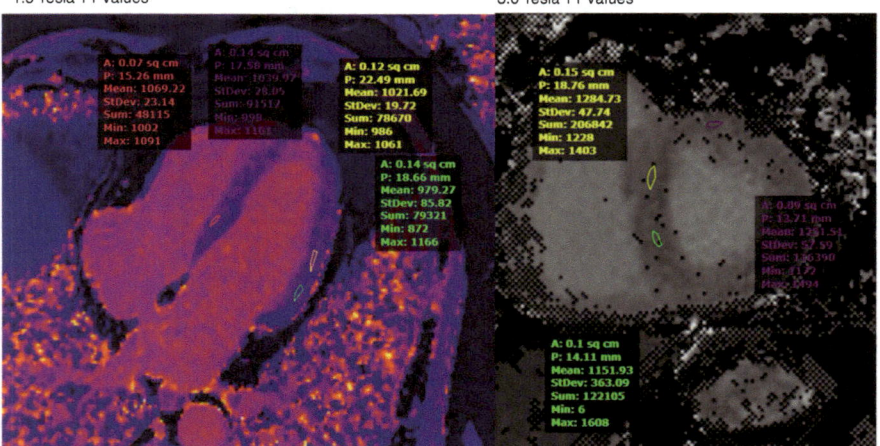

Native T1 Mapping On 1.5 Tesla

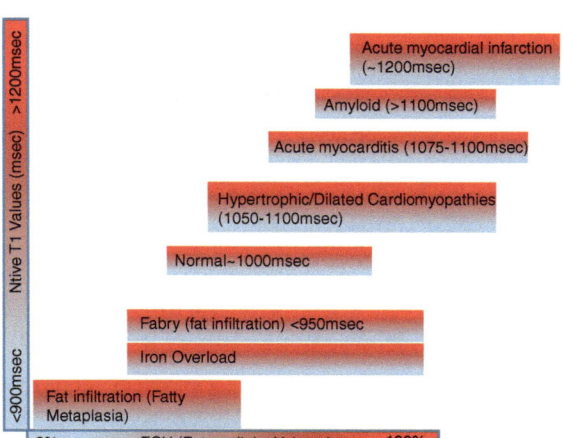

7. If a patient experiences cardiac arrest in the MRI. What is the next step?

(A) Begin CPR immediately
(B) Await the resuscitation team
(C) Press the Quench button and start resuscitation
(D) Pull patient from the MRI scanner, and immediately bring them to a lower zone, and begin resuscitation

The correct answer is D. While uncommon, cardiac arrest in the MRI scanner is a potential problem. Early assessment and recognition are key. If the patient becomes unresponsive, immediately remove the patient from the scan room, and bring them to the designated recovery area and call blue [12]. While it is tempting to begin CPR immediately, the potential for the code team to bring magnetic material and cause further harm in zone 4 is real, making A incorrect. Awaiting the resuscitation team is inappropriate in the ACLS algorithm. The quench button is only to be pressed if the patient is being crushed by a magnetic object, as the release of toxic gasses can risk asphyxiation.

8. A patient is undergoing a regadenoson stress test and begins to experience chest pain, the next step is:

(A) Immediately terminate the scan and bring patient to the recovery area
(B) Deliver nitroglycerin
(C) Continue with image acquisition
(D) Give aminophylline and terminate the scan

The correct answer is C. While it is tempting to terminate the scan or give aminophylline immediately, it is best to obtain images and then give aminophylline [13]. This is similar to the guidelines regarding nuclear stress tests. Terminating the scan immediately is inappropriate as long as there are no life-threatening arrhythmias, it is reasonable to proceed. Delivering nitroglycerin is incorrect as this chest pain will be limited. Giving aminophylline can occur after images are obtained, as giving aminophylline prematurely will make the images void.

9. A 25-year-old G1P1 woman was referred for cardiac MRI for evaluation of myocarditis. She is breastfeeding her infant. What would be the recommendation regarding breastfeeding after gadolinium administration?

(A) Pump and dump for 24 h
(B) Pump and dump for 48 h
(C) Pump and dump for 36 h
(D) Continue without interruption

The best choice answer is D. The 2022 ACR guidelines recommend continuation of breastfeeding as the amount of gadolinium that is excreted in milk and absorbed by the infant's gut is extremely low [14, 15]. A shared decision-making is important in these situations. Pregnant women, on the other hand, should avoid gadolinium at all costs possible due to pregnancy class C [16].

10. A steel mill factory worker presents for an outpatient MRI. The next step is to:

(A) Obtain permission from the prescribing physician
(B) Obtain orbital X-ray
(C) Head, neck, and chest CT
(D) Proceed with MRI

The correct answer is D. MRI in patients with occupations that increase their risk for having orbital metallic fragment is somewhat controversial [17], but believed mere occupational exposure to metal fragments is insufficient to warrant radiographic workup [18]. If there is suspicion that an orbital fragment is present or the patient is unclear, then orbital X-rays or head CT is recommended [19].

11. A patient presents for an MRI and says he has a retained bullet fragment in his neck but swears he has had prior scans with "no problem." The next logical step is:

(A) Obtain permission from the prescribing physician
(B) Obtain neck X-ray
(C) Chest CT
(D) Proceed with MRI

The correct answer is B. Patients with prior metallic foreign bodies are difficult [20]. Summary recommendations say that if the composition/location/shape is unknown to obtain X-ray prior to MRI [21].

12. The following delayed enhancement inversion recovery (magnitude) image demonstrates:

Delayed MAG Imaging

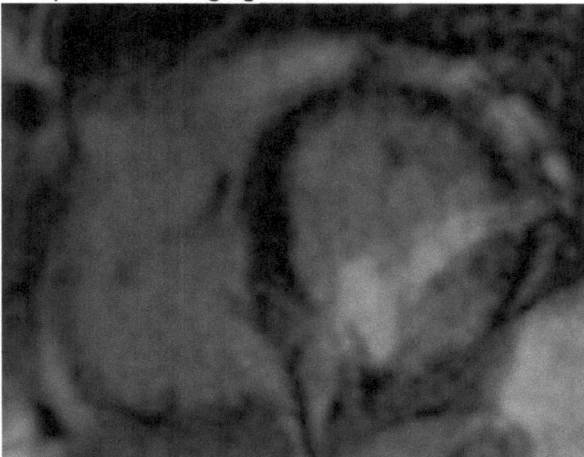

(A) Lateral wall infarct
(B) Anterior wall infarct
(C) Artifact
(D) Amyloidosis

The correct answer is C. The image demonstrates an artifact that obscures the lateral, inferior, and septal walls. The artifact also distorts some of the blood pool in addition to the myocardium. Artifacts typically occur in the phase encoding direction [22].

Delayed MAG Imaging

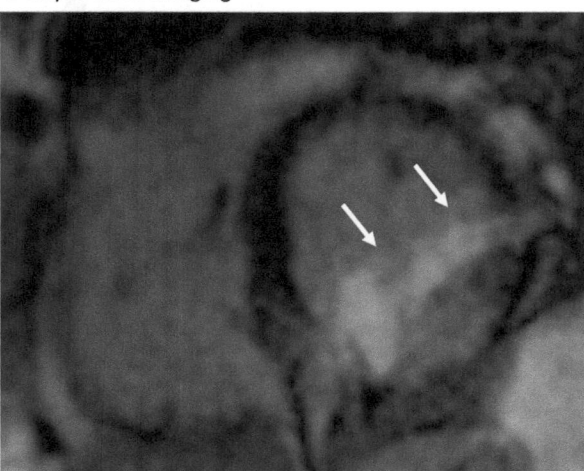

Delayed MAG Imaging with artifact
(white arrow) obscuring the
myocardium and blood pool

13. If we increase the acceleration factor of parallel imaging by a factor of 4, what
happens to the signal to noise ratio?

(A) Decreases to 50%
(B) Decreases to 60%
(C) Decreases to 71%
(D) Decreases to 95%

The correct answer is C. The equation relating parallel imaging SNR to acceleration factor is as follows:

$$\text{Parallel SNR} = \frac{\text{SNR}}{g\sqrt{R}}$$

where g is the geometry factor (constant) and R is the acceleration factor. In this
question, increasing the acceleration factor to 4 will result in a reduction of SNR to
$\frac{1}{\sqrt{2}}$ which is 0.71 [23].

14. What is the likely cause of this artifact?

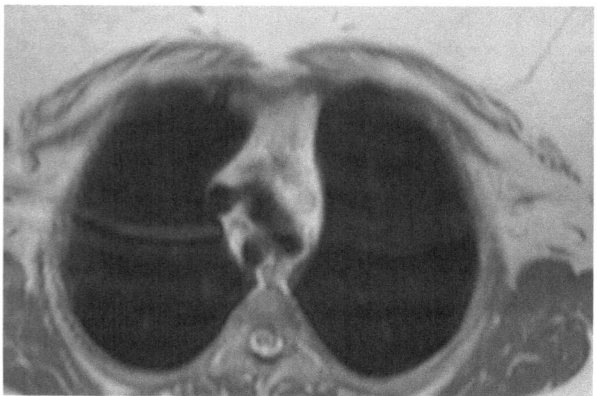

(A) Respiratory motion
(B) Arrhythmia
(C) Parallel imaging
(D) ECG gating artifact

The correct answer is A. The above image demonstrates an almost horizontal line
across the entire screen. This likely represents a respiratory motion artifact, which
typically occurs in the phase direction [24]. This can be corrected by changing
phase and frequency encoding, holding breathing. Using parallel imaging, you
decrease signal-to-noise ratio [25]. ECG gating artifacts result in rejected beats and
slightly jumpy images. Wrap/aliasing artifacts can also present similarly and can
contribute to the respiratory motion artifact when the chest moves anteriorly outside
the field of view.

HASTE Imaging

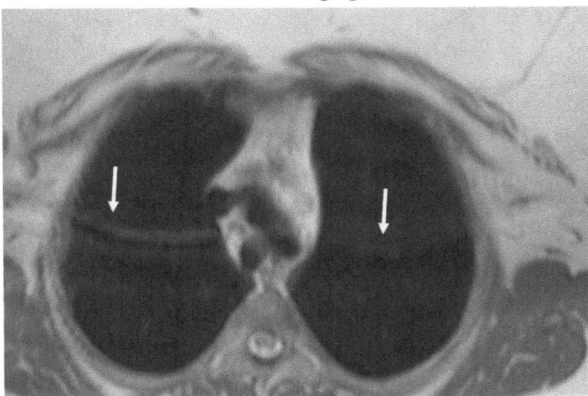

15. Which of the following sequences will cause the best suppression of fat?

(A) Spin echo
(B) Gradient echo
(C) Inversion recovery
(D) Phase contrast

The correct answer is C. Inversion recovery takes advantage of the difference in T1 recovery values of the tissue. The longitudinal magnetization of adipose will recover faster than water, so we can suppress the fat [26]. Gradient echo and spin echo are the normal imaging modalities for our cine and vascular imaging [27]. Phase contrast is used for velocity mapping [28].

16. In a patient with an ICD, before proceeding with the MRI, one must:

(A) Check chest X-ray prior
(B) Reprogram the device
(C) Place in asynchronous mode
(D) Monitor with continuous ECG/pulse oximetry
(E) A, B, C
(F) B, C, D

The correct answer is F. Prior to imaging patients with pacemakers/ICD, one needs to know the pacemaker model, pacemaker settings, reprogram the device, have an external defibrillator available outside zone 4, and monitor with continuous EKG [29]. Chest ray prior to MRI is no longer required unless there is a question of abandoned leads.

17. Which of the following is true regarding artifacts in patients with pacemakers?

(A) The artifact is often worse than in patients with ICD
(B) The artifact is reduced in MRI conditional devices compared with non-conditional devices

(C) The artifact is reduced with expiration
(D) The artifact is reduced by increasing the bandwidth
(E) The artifact is reduced with steady state-free precession imaging compared with Gradient Recall Echo

The correct answer is D. Increasing the bandwidth, single shot, motion-corrected images are best when large artifacts are caused by ICD or pacemakers. Wideband sequences are often used for delayed enhancement in patients with implanted devices. ICDs cause worse artifacts than pacemakers (due to larger equipment) so A is incorrect. Conditional vs non-conditional devices have not been shown to demonstrate impact on artifacts. Expiration will drop the chest and likely have the ICD closer to the field of view, which will make the artifact worse. Steady state-free precession is usually worse imaging than gradient echo in patients with ICD/pacemakers.

18. According to the American College of Radiology, MRI zone 1 is:

(A) The room containing the magnetic
(B) The waiting room for the open public
(C) Hallway leading to the scan room
(D) The control room

The correct answer is B. Zone 4 is the magnetic room and is an access restricted with no ferromagnetic devices allowed. Zone 1 is the check-in area for the general public [30].

19. In a 1.5-Tesla scanner, the difference between the number of spins aligned with as compared to the number of spins aligned against the main magnetic field is:

(A) 1 in 1,000,000,000
(B) 1 in 1,000,000
(C) 1 in 1,000
(D) 1 in 100

The correct answer is 1 in a 1,000,000. In a 1.5-Tesla scanner for every 2 million protons, about 5 more protons will be aligned with the field than against the field [31].

20. What does T1 time constant describe?

(A) Loss of longitudinal magnetization
(B) Loss of transverse magnetization
(C) Regrowth of longitudinal magnetization
(D) Regrowth of transverse magnetization

The correct answer is C. The T1 curve demonstrates regrowth of longitudinal magnetization. T2 relaxation represents the loss of transverse magnetization [32].

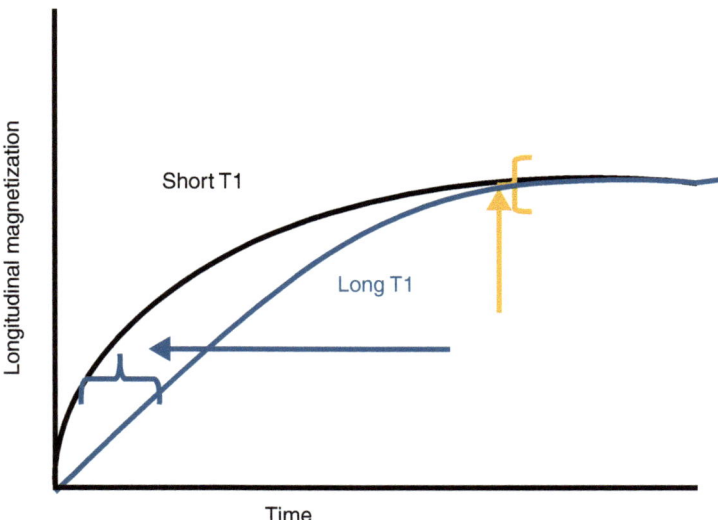

Blue arrow demonstrates larger
differentiation of tissues based on T1
compared to yellow arrow

21. All of the following have an application by CMR except:

(A) Imaging coronary artery aneurysm
(B) Identification of anomalous coronary arteries
(C) Identification of aortocoronary bypass grafts
(D) Assessment of coronary stenosis

The correct answer is D. Currently there is no clinical indication for CMR for assessment of coronary artery stenosis. While there are ongoing studies, this remains experimental and in the research phase. The rest of the choices all currently have indications for CMR imaging [33].

22. During a spin echo (SE) sequence, the time between the first and second radio frequency pulses is:

(A) TR
(B) TE
(C) TI
(D) TE/2

The correct answer is D. Spin echo occurs at time TE (echo time) which is exactly twice the inter-pulse spacing. TR is the repetition time, which is the time between 2 excitation pulses [34]. A single radiofrequency pulse creates free induction decay. The time between the first pulse and the peak of the spin echo is the echo time (TE).

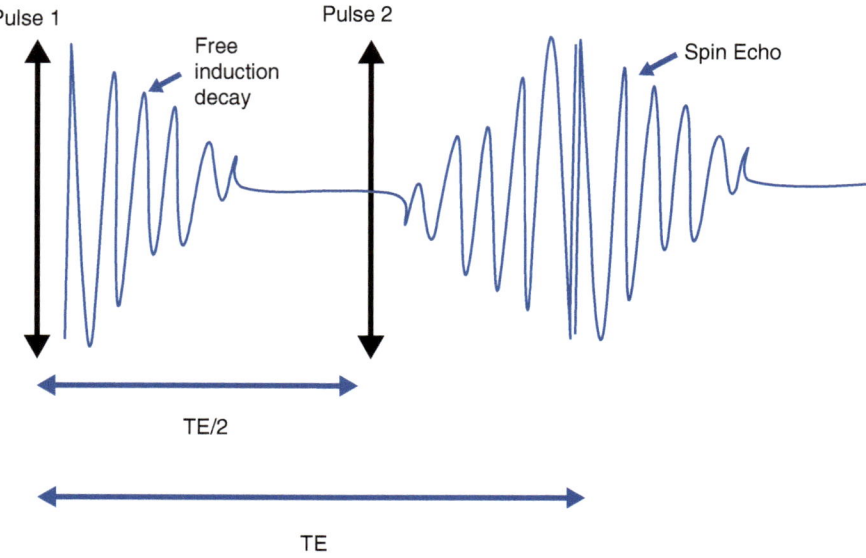

References

1. Ester A. Questions and answers in MRI. https://mriquestions.com/image-contrast-trte.html
2. Kawel-Boehm N, Hetzel SJ, Ambale-Venkatesh B, Captur G, Francois CJ, Jerosch-Herold M, Salerno M, Teague SD, Valsangiacomo-Buechel E, van der Geest RJ, Bluemke DA. Reference ranges ("normal values") for cardiovascular magnetic resonance (CMR) in adults and children: 2020 update. J Cardiovasc Magn Reson. 2020;22(1):87. https://doi.org/10.1186/s12968-020-00683-3.
3. Abi-Abdallah D, Robin V, Drochon A, Fokapu O. Alterations in human ECG due to the MagnetoHydroDynamic effect: a method for accurate R peak detection in the presence of high MHD artifacts. In: 2007 29th Annual International Conference of the IEEE Engineering in Medicine and Biology Society. IEEE, Lyon, France, 2007. p 1842–5.
4. Izgi C. MRI evaluation of aortic stenosis: flow evaluation. 2022. https://www.escardio.org/Education/Practice-Tools/EACVI-toolboxes/Valvular-Imaging/Atlas-of-valvular-imaging/MRI-evaluation-of-aortic-stenosis-flow-evaluation
5. Huang SY, Seethamraju RT, Patel P, Hahn PF, Kirsch JE, Guimaraes AR. Body MR imaging: artifacts, k-space, and solutions. RadioGraphics. 2015;35(5):1439–60. https://doi.org/10.1148/rg.2015140289.
6. Deshmane A, Gulani V, Griswold MA, Seiberlich N. Parallel MR imaging. J Magn Reson Imaging. 2012;36(1):55–72. https://doi.org/10.1002/jmri.23639.
7. International Electrotechnical Commission (IEC). Medical electrical equipment. Particular requirements for the safety of magnetic resonance equipment for medical diagnosis. Int Electrotechical Comm Int Stand 2010 IEC60601-2-33. 2010.
8. Frankel J, Wilén J, Hansson Mild K. Assessing exposures to magnetic resonance imaging's complex mixture of magnetic fields for in vivo, in vitro, and epidemiologic studies of health effects for staff and patients. Front Public Health. 2018;6:66. https://doi.org/10.3389/fpubh.2018.00066.

9. Haaf P, Garg P, Messroghli DR, Broadbent DA, Greenwood JP, Plein S. Cardiac T1 mapping and extracellular volume (ECV) in clinical practice: a comprehensive review. J Cardiovasc Magn Reson. 2017;18(1):89. https://doi.org/10.1186/s12968-016-0308-4.

10. Weingärtner S, Meßner NM, Budjan J, Loßnitzer D, Mattler U, Papavassiliu T, Zöllner FG, Schad LR. Myocardial T1-mapping at 3T using saturation-recovery: reference values, precision and comparison with MOLLI. J Cardiovasc Magn Reson. 2017;18(1):84. https://doi.org/10.1186/s12968-016-0302-x.

11. Thompson RB, Chow K, Khan A, Chan A, Shanks M, Paterson I, Oudit GY. Mapping with cardiovascular MRI is highly sensitive for fabry disease independent of hypertrophy and sex. Circ Cardiovasc Imaging. 2013;6(5):637–45. https://doi.org/10.1161/CIRCIMAGING.113.000482.

12. UCSF Radiology. cMRI Code Blue Protocol. In: UCSF Dep. Radiol. 2022. https://radiology.ucsf.edu/patient-care/patient-safety/mri/code-blue. Accessed 28 Aug 2022.

13. Elkholy KO, Hegazy O, Okunade A, Aktas S, Ajibawo T. Regadenoson stress testing: a comprehensive review with a focused update. Cureus. 2021. https://doi.org/10.7759/cureus.12940

14. ACR Committee On Drugs and Contrast ACR Manual on Contrast Media 2022. Am Coll Radiol.

15. Webb JAW, Thomsen HS, Morcos SK, Members of Contrast Media Safety Committee of European Society of Urogenital Radiology (ESUR). The use of iodinated and gadolinium contrast media during pregnancy and lactation. Eur Radiol. 2005;15(6):1234–40. https://doi.org/10.1007/s00330-004-2583-y.

16. Oh K, Roberts V, Schabel M. Gadolinium chelate contrast material in pregnancy: fetal biodistribution in the nonhuman primate. Radiology. 2015;276(1):110–8.

17. Elster A. Phase-contrast MRA. In: MRI quest. https://mriquestions.com/phase-contrast-mra.html. Accessed 10 Jun 2022.

18. Jarvik, JG, Ramsey S. Radiographic screening for orbital foreign bodies prior to MR imaging: is it worth it? AJNR AM J Neuroradiol.

19. Otto PM, Otto RA, Virapongse C, Friedman SM, Emerson S, Li KCP, Malot R, Kaude JV, Staab EV. Screening test for detection of metallic foreign objects in the orbit before magnetic resonance imaging. Invest Radiol. 1992;27(4):308–10. https://doi.org/10.1097/00004424-199204000-00010.

20. Elster Orbital Foreign Bodies. https://mriquestions.com/orbital-foreign-bodies.html

21. Jabehdar Maralani P, Schieda N, Hecht EM, Litt H, Hindman N, Heyn C, Davenport MS, Zaharchuk G, Hess CP, Weinreb J. MRI safety and devices: an update and expert consensus. J Magn Reson Imaging. 2020;51(3):657–74. https://doi.org/10.1002/jmri.26909.

22. Morelli JN, Runge VM, Ai F, Attenberger U, Vu L, Schmeets SH, Nitz WR, Kirsch JE. An image-based approach to understanding the physics of MR artifacts. RadioGraphics. 2011;31(3):849–66. https://doi.org/10.1148/rg.313105115.

23. Elster A. Using parallel imaging. https://mriquestions.com/why-and-when-to-use.html

24. Honal M, Leupold J, Huff S, Baumann T, Ludwig U. Compensation of breathing motion artifacts for MRI with continuously moving table: breathing motion compensation for CMT-MRI. Magn Reson Med. 2010;63(3):701–12. https://doi.org/10.1002/mrm.22162.

25. Dietrich O, Raya JG, Reeder SB, Reiser MF, Schoenberg SO. Measurement of signal-to-noise ratios in MR images: influence of multichannel coils, parallel imaging, and reconstruction filters. J Magn Reson Imaging. 2007;26(2):375–85. https://doi.org/10.1002/jmri.20969.

26. Delfaut EM, Beltran J, Johnson G, Rousseau J, Marchandise X, Cotten A. Fat suppression in MR imaging: techniques and pitfalls. RadioGraphics. 1999;19(2):373–82. https://doi.org/10.1148/radiographics.19.2.g99mr03373.

27. Ridgway JP. Cardiovascular magnetic resonance physics for clinicians: part I. J Cardiovasc Magn Reson. 2010;12(1):71. https://doi.org/10.1186/1532-429X-12-71.

28. Biglands JD, Radjenovic A, Ridgway JP. Cardiovascular magnetic resonance physics for clinicians: part II. J Cardiovasc Magn Reson. 2012;14(1):66. https://doi.org/10.1186/1532-429X-14-66.

29. Kodali S, Baher A, Shah D. Safety of MRIs in patients with pacemakers and defibrillators. Methodist DeBakey Cardiovasc J. 2013;9(3):137. https://doi.org/10.14797/mdcj-9-3-137.
30. UCSF Radiology. Access restriction. In: Access restrict. 2022. https://radiology.ucsf.edu/patient-care/patient-safety/mri/access-restriction. Accessed 28 Aug 2022.
31. NessAiver M. Simply physics the home of MRI physics put simply. In: Simply Phys. 2022. http://www.simplyphysics.com/page2_2.html. Accessed 28 Aug 2022.
32. An H, Lin W. Spin density T1, T2, and T2* relaxation and Bloch equations. Curr Protoc Magn Reson Imaging. 2001;00(1) https://doi.org/10.1002/0471142719.mib0301s00.
33. Pennell D. Clinical indications for cardiovascular magnetic resonance (CMR): consensus panel report? Eur Heart J. 2004;25(21):1940–65. https://doi.org/10.1016/j.ehj.2004.06.040.
34. Elster A. MRI questions. In: Spin Echo. https://mriquestions.com/spin-echo1.html

Chapter 2
Patient-Specific Protocols

23. How does one contour to calculate left ventricular ejection fraction and myocardial mass?

(A) Left Ventricle endomyocardial outlines
(B) LV epicardial and endomyocardial outlines
(C) LV epicardial outlines
(D) Left ventricle epicardial, endomyocardial, and aortic valve velocity

The correct answer is B. To calculate left ventricular stroke volume, left ventricle endomyocardial outlines need to be performed. To calculate left ventricular myocardial mass, left ventricle epicardial outlines need to be additionally contoured in diastole. The aortic valve velocity is needed for mitral regurgitation, but not LV ejection fraction or LV myocardial mass [1].

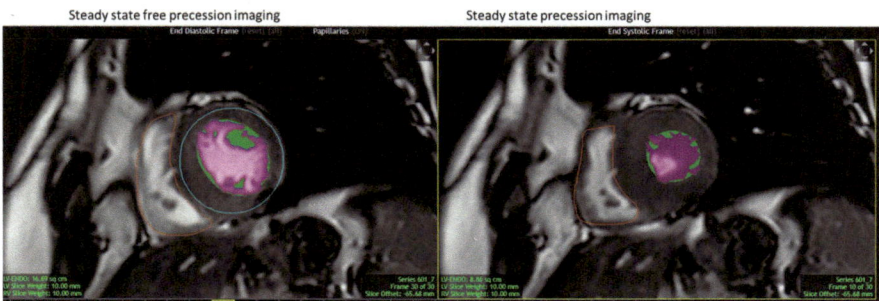

Demonstrating epicardial contour for LV mass calculation. Red arrow demonstrating endomyocardial contour.

17

S. G. Al-Kindi, S. E. Janus, *Cardiac MRI Certification Exam*, https://doi.org/10.1007/978-3-031-25966-1_2

24. A patient with severe asthma and second-degree heart block presents for a stress MRI. The next best step is?

(A) Proceed with regadenoson stress
(B) Proceed with adenosine stress
(C) Proceed with dobutamine stress
(D) Proceed with dipyridamole stress

The correct answer is C. Adenosine and to a lesser extent regadenoson are contraindicated in second-degree heart block. Dipyridamole is contraindicated to significant reactive airway disease, systolic blood pressure >200 mmHg or <90 mmHg, and caffeine intake in prior 12 h [2]. So, dobutamine is the only option remaining.

25. A patient presents for an outpatient stress test with an audible wheeze. Despite nebulizers, the wheeze remains. How do you proceed next?

(A) Proceed with regadenoson stress
(B) Proceed with adenosine stress
(C) Proceed with dipyridamole stress
(D) Cancel the exam and reschedule

The correct answer is D. The best option would be to cancel the exam and reschedule. Dobutamine is allowed in asthma/wheeze, it is not an option here. So, the next best choice is to reschedule the elective case [3]. Adenosine and to a lesser extent regadenoson are contraindicated in an active wheeze. Dipyridamole is contraindicated in significant reactive airway disease.

26. How do you correct this delayed enhancement image?

PSIR Delayed enhancement imaging

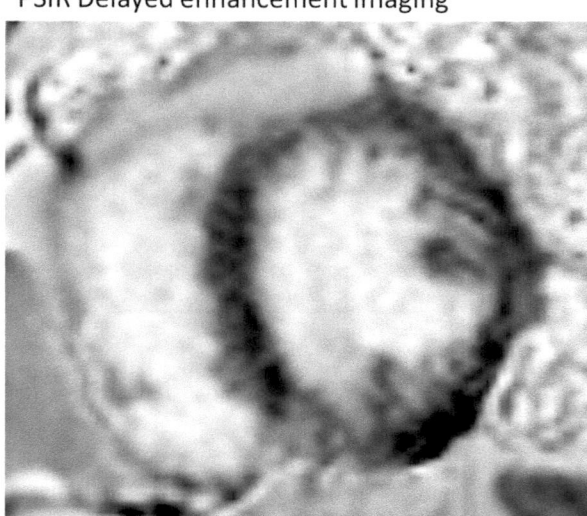

(A) Lengthen TI time
(B) Shorten TI time
(C) Change frequency and phase encoding
(D) Change flip angle

The correct answer is A, i.e., lengthen the TI time. As seen below, an early TI time will not correctly null the myocardium and the blood pool will not show good differentiation [4]. A late TI time will cause the myocardium to no longer be nulled. The TI time must be continuously increased during late enhancement scanning.

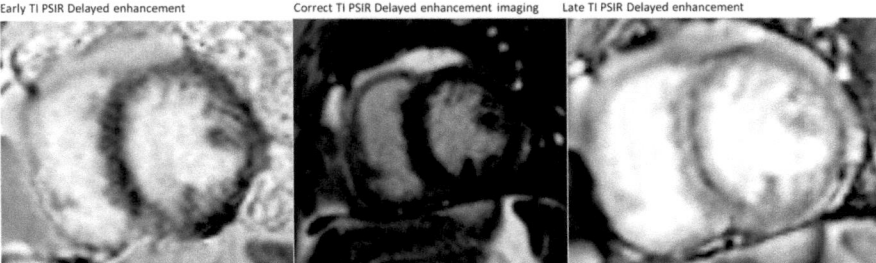

Early TI PSIR Delayed enhancement   Correct TI PSIR Delayed enhancement imaging   Late TI PSIR Delayed enhancement

Delayed enhancement imaging shows an incorrect TI time with the TI time being set too early. The null point of the myocardium is not achieved correctly. On the middle image the TI is correctly chosen and the myocardium is nulled. On right image, TI time is too late resulting in incorrect nulling of the myocardium.

27. A patient with a pacemaker is brought to be scanned for cardiac MRI, which of the following is an inappropriate pacemaker setting?

(A) VOO
(B) DOO
(C) AOO single lead
(D) DDD

The correct answer is D. Choices A, B, and C are all asynchronous pacing modes, which are appropriate. Option D demonstrates dual chamber paced, dual chamber sensed, and still has inhibition turned on. When scanning patients with ICD, one wished to use an asynchronous pacing mode [5].

28. What happens by sampling only the periphery of K space?

(A) Increase contrast
(B) Increase shape
(C) Decrease contrast
(D) Decrease spatial resolution

The correct answer is C. The center of K space contains low frequencies (basic contrast, shapes). The peripheral of K space contains details and edges. Therefore, MR angiography, for example, takes advantage of sampling only the center of K space [6] which allows short scan time, with low spatial resolution and good contrast.

29. When is the time to trigger for imaging of the coronary flow?

ECG Gating

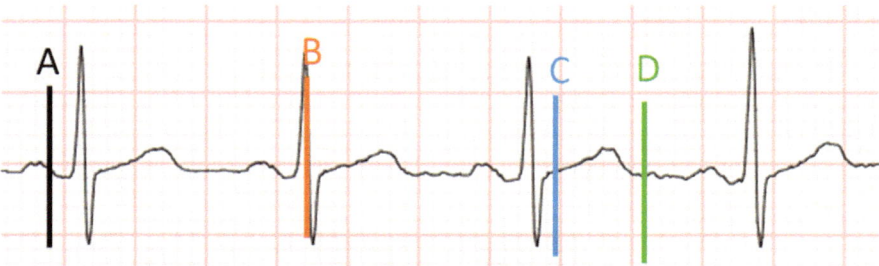

(A) A
(B) B
(C) C
(D) D

    The correct answer is D. To image coronary flow early diastole is the correct time [7]. Early diastole occurs after the T wave, so choice D is the correct answer.

30. What is the correct interpretation of these stress images?

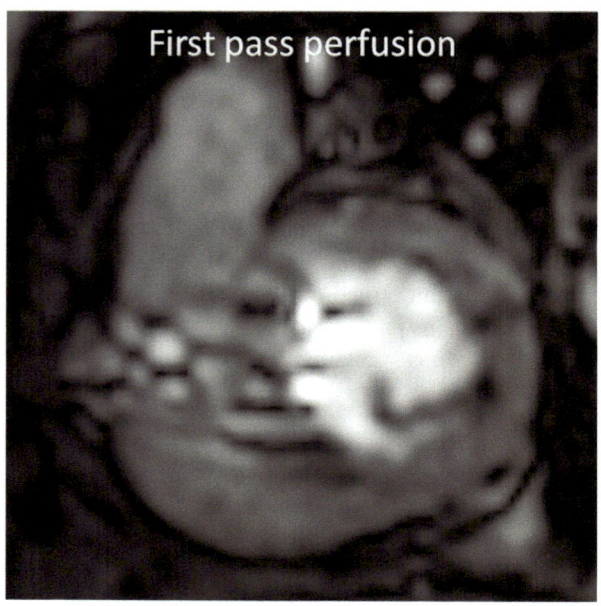

First pass perfusion

(A) Anterior wall ischemia
(B) Inferior wall ischemia
(C) Lateral wall ischemia
(D) Septal wall ischemia
(E) Artifact

The answer is E. There is an artifact in the septal and lateral walls that runs through the entire image including the myocardium [8].

31. Artifacts are most commonly seen in:

(A) The phase encoding direction
(B) The frequency encoding direction
(C) The B0 gradient field
(D) The oblique angels

The correct answer is A. Artifacts most commonly are seen in the phase encoding direction due to prolonged signal acquisition time in that direction, but can happen in any direction [9].

32. All of the following are ways to reduce scan time except:

(A) Increase parallel imaging
(B) Decrease phase encoding
(C) Increase data lines per cycle
(D) Multiple acquisitions

The correct answer is D. Multiple acquisitions (like Cine imaging, or increasing Number of excitations (NEX)) actually require more time to obtain. By increasing parallel imaging we decrease scan time [10] but also decrease signal to noise ratio [11]. Decreasing phase encoding lines decreases scan time, increases signal to noise ratio, but decreases spatial resolution. Increasing the data lines per cell, decreases scan time, but increases cardiac motion artifacts.

33. All of the following are ways to minimize wrap artifact except:

(A) Increase the field of view
(B) Oversampling
(C) Under sampling
(D) Correct B0 inhomogeneities

The correct answer is D. B0 inhomogeneities are a disruption in the main magnetic field [12]. This causes signal loss or image distortion and is rectified with localized shimming or applying different metallic pieces to the scanner. This has nothing to do with wrap artifact. Wrap artifacts can be minimized by increasing the field of view (will increase signal to noise ratio, decrease spatial resolution), oversampling (increase scan time, increase signal to noise ratio), or under sampling (decrease signal to noise, decrease scan time).

34. What is the most likely cause of this artifact?

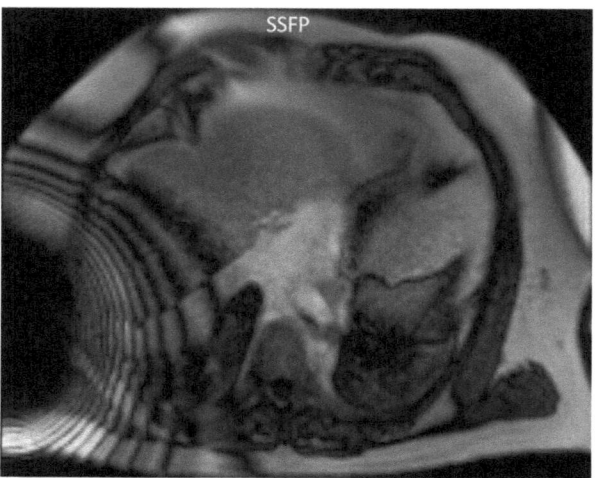

(A) ICD artifact
(B) Metal external to the patient
(C) Radio being played in Zone 3
(D) Zone 4 door left open

The correct answer is B. This is a typical large pattern of artifact located solely on one side of the body due to a metallic object outside the body (e.g., hearing aids and car keys in pocket) [13]. ICD artifacts would occur typically in the left upper chest (left-sided devices) or less likely in the right chest. Radio being played in zone 3 or the door being left open will cause a zipper artifact [14].

35. Which of the following are contraindications to MRI?

(A) Pregnancy
(B) Breastfeeding
(C) Leadless pacemaker
(D) Retained pacemaker leads after extraction of generator

The correct answer is D. Abandoned pacemaker/ICD leads remain a contraindication to MRI, although emerging data suggest that it might be safe to scan these patients [15]. Other absolute contraindications are left ventricular assist device, metallic foreign body in the eye, insulin pumps, and temporary transvenous pacing leads [16]. Pregnancy is a relative contraindication to gadolinium. Breastfeeding is no longer a contraindication to gadolinium. Leadless pacemakers (Micra© devices) are MRI conditional [17].

36. What is the correct definition of MPR and MIP?

(A) Multi-plane reconstitution/Maximum Projection Intensity
(B) Multiple-iterative reconstruction/Many Images Projection
(C) Multiple planar reconstruction/ Maximum Projection Intensity
(D) Maximum projection intensity/Multi-plane reconstitution
(E) None of the above

   The correct answer is C. MPR stands for multiple planar reconstruction [18]. It allows the ability to obtain orthogonal views to truly become perpendicular to a structure. MIP stands for maximum projection intensity and consists of projecting a voxel with the highest attenuation value onto the 2D image being viewed [19]. Iterative reconstruction is reconstruction of raw data using a filtered back projection system [20].

37. What is the most likely diagnosis on this perfusion image after regadenoson administration?

First Pass Perfusion

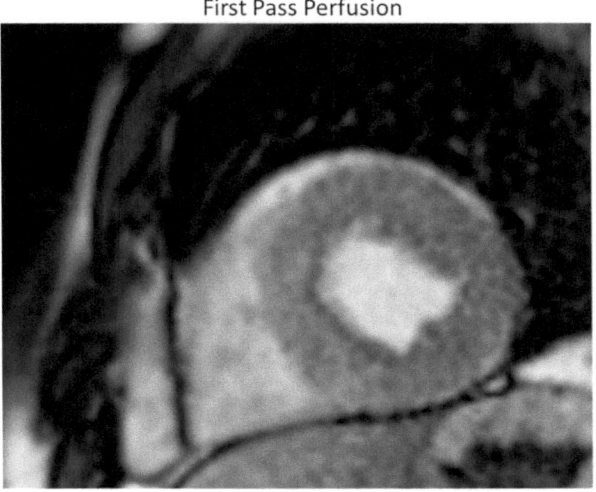

(A) Ischemia in the anterior wall
(B) Ischemia in the septal wall
(C) Ischemia in the inferior wall
(D) Artifact
(E) Multi-vessel disease

   The correct answer is D. The above image demonstrates dark rim artifact at the interaction between contrast (bright) and non-contrast (dark) rim, leading to an artifact [21]. Compared to ischemia which would be more than one voxel and permanent, this artifact is usually temporary and in the phase encoding direction, but can also occur in the frequency encoding direction.

First Pass Perfusion

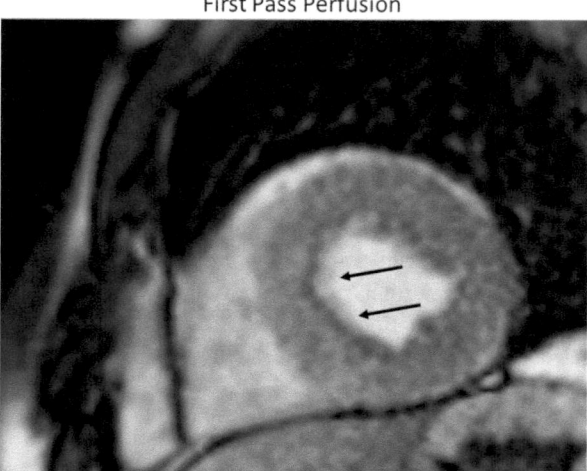

First Pass Perfusion- demonstrating dark rim artifact.
Believed to be due to susceptibility from the
gadolinium bolus, motion and/or resolution art he
interface.

38. Potential ways to reduce ICD artifacts include all of the following except:

(A) Imaging during inspiration
(B) Wideband pulse sequences
(C) FLASH sequences
(D) Avoiding sequences like turbo spin

The answer is D. Turbo spin echo is a good sequence to use to reduce ICD artifact. Imaging during inspiration will lower the diaphragm and move the ICD further away from the heart. Flash sequences also help reduce ICD artifacts [22].

FFSP- Real time   FSSP- Inspiration

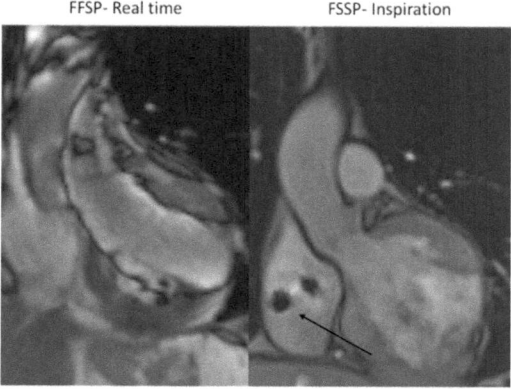

Inspiration lowering the diaphragm and reducing the artifact from
the ICD (black arrow)

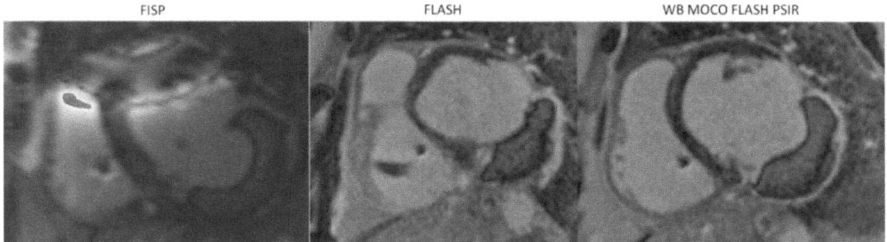

Flash and wide band flash with motion correction (MOCO) demonstrating improved ability to discern images in patients with ICDs or pacemakers

39. Name the artifact?

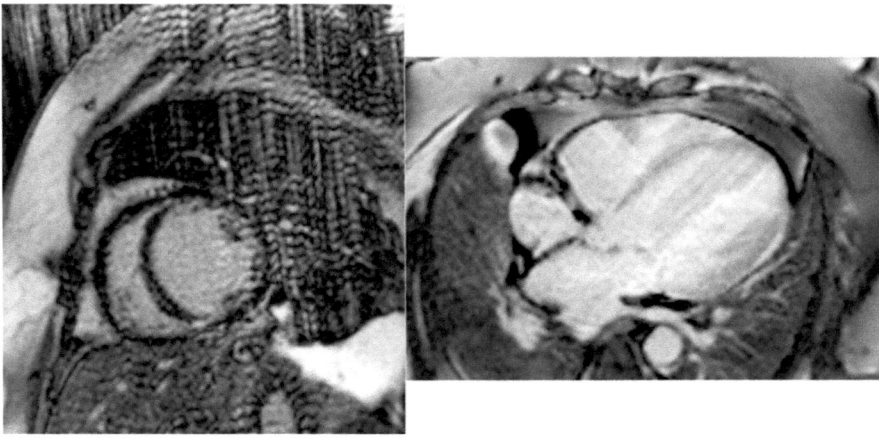

(A) Aliasing/Wrap around
(B) B0 inhomogeneity
(C) Susceptibility artifacts
(D) Herringbone artifact

This is likely a Herringbone artifact. Herringbone artifact involves electromagnetic spikes and can occur in any direction or one or multiple images. Herringbone artifact is usually related to aberrant data points in K space. The regularly striped pattern resembling fabric is the classic pattern [23].

40. To create spin echo, one applies:

(A) Reverse the field of direction of B0
(B) Add shimming magnets
(C) Create saturation from fat
(D) Apply a flip using a second radiofrequency pulse

The correct answer is D. To create a spin echo or a train of echos, one applies a flip using a second radiofrequency pulse (usually 180 degrees) [24]. Using multiple spin echos can create a train of echo length to fill K space faster like in HASTE imaging (half-acquired turbo spin echo). Reversing the field direction of B0 will only change the longitudinal magnetization vector [25]. Adding shimming magnets gets rid of inhomogeneity in the main field. Inversion recovery or fat suppression nulls the fat to better achieve water/fat difference [26].

41. To assess for edema post-myocardial infarction, which series would give best/ most complete evaluation?

(A) T2 mapping, T2* mapping, T1W Late gadolinium imaging
(B) T2 mapping, STIR, early gadolinium imaging
(C) T1 mapping, T2* mapping, Early gadolinium imaging
(D) T1 mapping, STIR, T1-weighted imaging

The correct answer is A. The recommended is for tissue characterization including mapping techniques like T2 mapping, T2*, and T1W LGE. T2 provides information on myocardial edema, while T2* provides information on infarct hemorrhage. LGE provides information on the size of the infarction and area at risk. T2-weighted imaging (e.g., STIR) can be helpful, but not recommended and may miss hemorrhage. T2W bright blood is not helpful for small NSTEMI. Early gadolinium imaging is helpful for thrombus and edema.

42. When imaging coronary arteries with elevated heart rates (>110 beats per minute), the best time to scan would be?

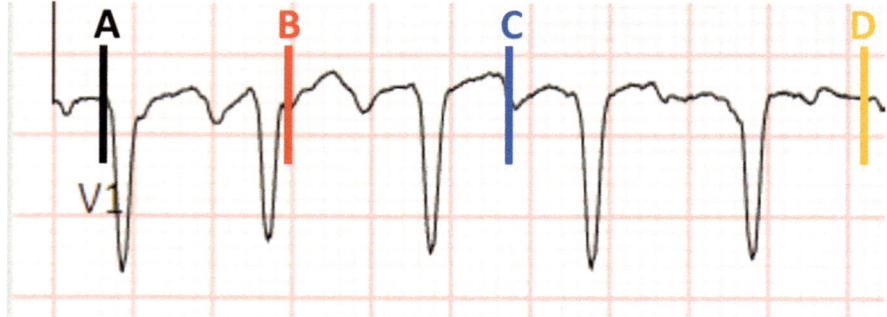

(A) A
(B) B
(C) C
(D) D

The correct answer is C at the end systole. When heart rate becomes elevated the diastolic period shortens. Therefore, it is best to image at the end systole or the end of the T Wave. A demonstrates beginning of systole. B is mid-systole. D is early/ mid-diastole.

43. Gradient recall echo has the following advances over steady state precession, except:

(A) GRE has worse signal to noise ratio
(B) GRE has worse contrast to noise ratio
(C) GRE has better ability with metal/valvular artifacts
(D) GRE has a better ability with fat-water artifact

The correct answer is D. Gradient recall echo has worse signal to noise ratio [27], worse contrast to noise, and worse fat-water artifact than SSFP. Gradient echo is useful for magnetic field and metal artifacts. Therefore, the only answer that is not true to D.

44. What is the best way to reduce this artifact and optimize the delayed enhancement imaging?

FISP

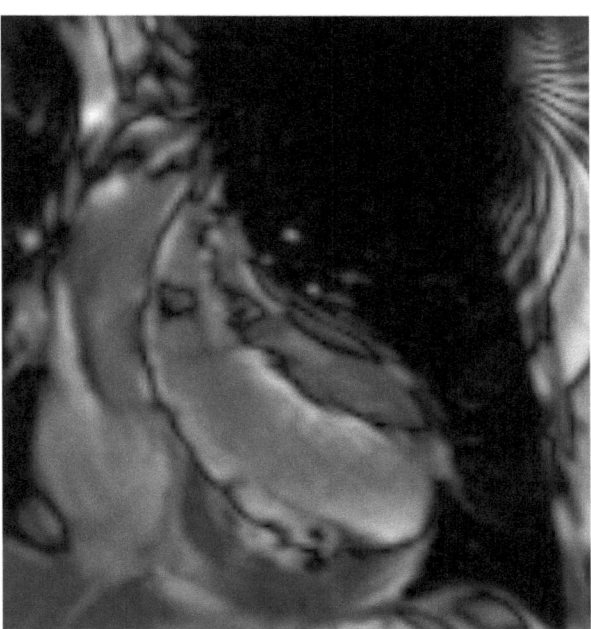

(A) Continue FISP as best series for ICDs
(B) Change to FLASH series
(C) Change to wide band imaging
(D) Change to Wide band with FLASH

The correct answer is D. Artifacts from ICDs are common. Ways to improve imaging to include FLASH, wide band series, motion correction, on delayed imaging [28]. By using all these in combination will provide the best possible imaging for delayed enhancement series.

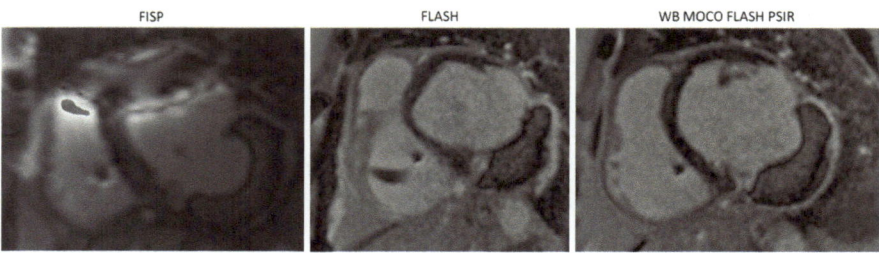

45. In patients with variable rhythms like atrial fibrillation, the best way to gate would be:

(A) Retrospective gating
(B) Prospective gating
(C) Real-time imaging
(D) Pulse gating

The correct answer is B, prospective gating. For the vast majority of patients, retrospective gating is the correct answer. Retrospective gating is the most commonly used when you have a clear ECG signal with good breath hold [29]. However, retrospective gating may miss the full cardiac cycle when there is frequency ectopy or variable R-R interval. Therefore, for patients with variable rhythms prospective gating is better as the systolic phase is generally unchanged [30].

Retrospective Gating

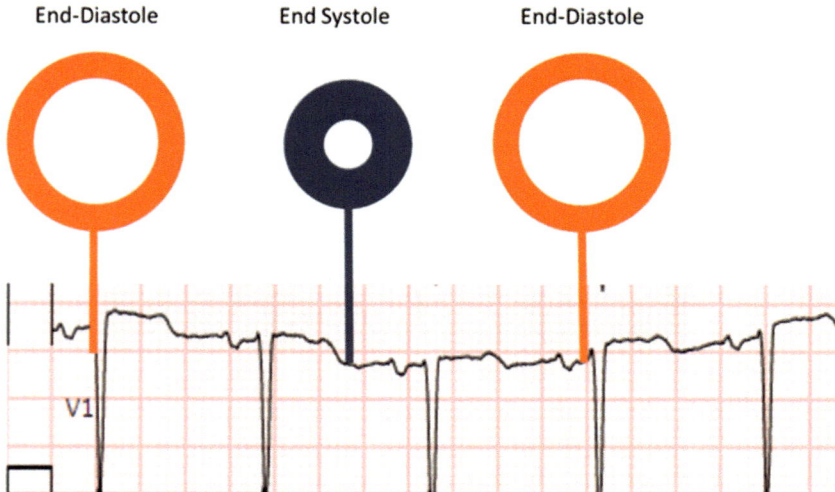

Prospective Gating

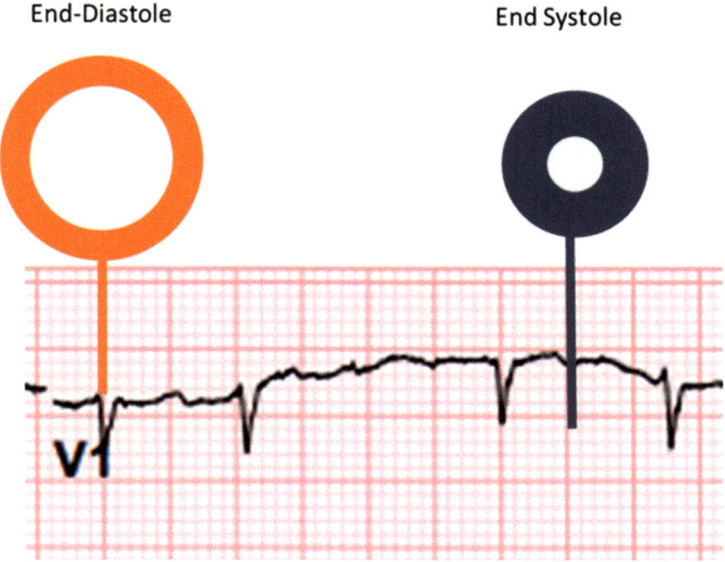

46. Parallel imaging decreases signal to noise ratio, but allows:

(A) Increased spatial resolution
(B) Reduce susceptibility artifact
(C) Increased reconstructed field of view
(D) Decreasing the scan time

The correct answer is D. Parallel imaging decreases scan time. Parallel imaging produces less phase encoding lines to be acquired over the same span of K space, making less time to acquire an image without changing spatial resolution [10].

47. You are completing a regadenoson stress test. The patient complains of shortness of breath and palpitations after injection. The telemetry shows Mobitz type II second-degree block which is new from prior first-degree AV block with a heart rate of 30 and blood pressure of 100/50 mmHg.

(A) Give aminophylline and re-evaluate
(B) Begin CPR
(C) Insert emergent temporary venous pacemaker
(D) Transcutaneous pace

The correct answer is A. The patient demonstrates hemodynamic stability despite being in Mobitz II [31]. Give aminophylline and await. You should only begin CPR and if the there was a loss of pulse [32]. Inserting invasive lines is not recommended if a temporary heart block is iatrogenic and potentially transient.

48. A 52-year-old man presents with myocardial infarction and undergoes coronary angiography that shows multi-vessel disease. A cardiac MRI is ordered to assess viability. When is the recommended time for MRI to assess infarct size?

(A) 24 h
(B) 48 h
(C) 5 ± 2 days
(D) 14 days

The correct answer is 5 ± 2 days [33]. Recommended due to healing of the myocardium. In the acute setting, LGE can represent both infarction and myocardial edema. At 5 ± 2 days, the edema improves and what remains is the infarction which correlates with imaging findings at 3 months. Imaging at 14 days would provide equivalent information on infarct size but requires an unnecessary delay.

References

1. Suinesiaputra A, Bluemke DA, Cowan BR, Friedrich MG, Kramer CM, Kwong R, Plein S, Schulz-Menger J, Westenberg JJM, Young AA, Nagel E. Quantification of LV function and mass by cardiovascular magnetic resonance: multi-center variability and consensus contours. J Cardiovasc Magn Reson. 2015;17(1):63. https://doi.org/10.1186/s12968-015-0170-9.
2. Pagnanelli RA, Camposano HL. Pharmacologic stress testing with myocardial perfusion imaging. J Nucl Med Technol. 2017;45(4):249–52. https://doi.org/10.2967/jnmt.117.199208.
3. Elhendy A, Bax JJ, Poldermans D. Dobutamine stress myocardial perfusion imaging in coronary artery disease. J Nucl Med 29.
4. Pandey T, Jambhekar K, Shaikh R, Lensing S, Viswamitra S. Utility of the inversion scout sequence (TI scout) in diagnosing myocardial amyloid infiltration. Int J Cardiovasc Imaging. 2013;29(1):103–12. https://doi.org/10.1007/s10554-012-0042-4.
5. Klein-Wiele O, Garmer M, Barbone G, Urbien R, Busch M, Kara K, Schäfer H, Schulte-Hermes M, Hailer B, Grönemeyer D. Deactivation vs. asynchronous pacing - prospective evaluation of a protocol for rhythm management in patients with magnetic resonance conditional pacemakers undergoing adenosine stress cardiovascular magnetic resonance imaging. BMC Cardiovasc Disord. 2017;17(1):142. https://doi.org/10.1186/s12872-017-0579-1.
6. Mezrich R. A perspective on K-space. Radiology. 1995;195(2):297–315. https://doi.org/10.1148/radiology.195.2.7724743.
7. Azarine A, Garçon P, Stansal A, Canepa N, Angelopoulos G, Silvera S, Sidi D, Marteau V, Zins M. Four-dimensional flow MRI: principles and cardiovascular applications. RadioGraphics. 2019;39(3):632–48. https://doi.org/10.1148/rg.2019180091.
8. Ferreira PF, Gatehouse PD, Mohiaddin RH, Firmin DN. Cardiovascular magnetic resonance artefacts. J Cardiovasc Magn Reson. 2013;15(1):41. https://doi.org/10.1186/1532-429X-15-41.
9. Elster A. Choosing PE & FE directions. https://mriquestions.com/choosing-pefe-direction.html#:~:text=The%20phase%2Dencoding%20direction%20is,in%20the%20phase%2Dencode%20direction. Accessed 10 Jun 2022.
10. Deshmane A, Gulani V, Griswold MA, Seiberlich N. Parallel MR imaging. J Magn Reson Imaging. 2012;36(1):55–72. https://doi.org/10.1002/jmri.23639.
11. George R. Signal to Noise Ratio. https://mrimaster.com/technique%20SNR.html. Accessed 10 Jun 2022.
12. Digma LA, Feng CH, Conlin CC, Rodríguez-Soto AE, Zhong AY, Hussain TS, Lui AJ, Batra K, Simon AB, Karunamuni R, Kuperman J, Rakow-Penner R, Hahn ME, Dale AM, Seibert

TM. Correcting B0 inhomogeneity-induced distortions in whole-body diffusion MRI of bone. Sci Rep. 2022;12(1):265. https://doi.org/10.1038/s41598-021-04467-2.

13. Bekiesińska-Figatowska M. Artifacts in magnetic resonance imaging. Pol J Radiol. 2015;80:93–106. https://doi.org/10.12659/PJR.892628.

14. Gaillard F. Zipper artifact. https://radiopaedia.org/articles/zipper-artifact?lang=us. Accessed 10 Jun 2022.

15. Schaller R. Magnetic resonance imaging in patients with cardiac implantable electronic devices with abandoned leads cardiology. JAMA Cardiol. 2021. https://doi.org/10.1001/jamacardio.2020.7572

16. Levine G, Gomes A. Safety of magnetic resonance imaging in patients with cardiovascular devices. Circulation. 2007;116(24):2878–91.

17. Soejima K. Safety evaluation of a leadless transcatheter pacemaker for magnetic resonance imaging use. Heart Rhythm. 2016;10:2056–63. https://doi.org/10.1016/j.hrthm.2016.06.032.

18. Bell D. Multiplanar reformation (MPR). In: Radiopaedia. https://radiopaedia.org/articles/multiplanar-reformation-mpr?lang=us. Accessed 10 Jun 2022.

19. Murphy A Maximum intensity projection. In: Radiopaedia. https://radiopaedia.org/articles/maximum-intensity-projection?lang=us. Accessed 10 Jun 2022.

20. Shuman W. Iterative reconstruction in CT: what does it do? How can I use it? In: Image Wisely. 2016. https://www.imagewisely.org/Imaging-Modalities/Computed-Tomography/Iterative-Reconstruction-in-CT. Accessed 10 Jun 2022.

21. Di Bella EVR, Parker DL, Sinusas AJ. On the dark rim artifact in dynamic contrast-enhanced MRI myocardial perfusion studies. Magn Reson Med. 2005;54(5):1295–9. https://doi.org/10.1002/mrm.20666.

22. Bhuva AN, Treibel TA, Seraphim A, Scully P, Knott KD, Augusto JB, Torlasco C, Menacho K, Lau C, Patel K, Moon JC, Kellman P, Manisty CH. Measurement of T1 mapping in patients with cardiac devices: off-resonance error extends beyond visual artifact but can be quantified and corrected. Front Cardiovasc Med. 2021;8:631366. https://doi.org/10.3389/fcvm.2021.631366.

23. Gaillard F. Herringbone artifact. In: Radiopaedia. https://radiopaedia.org/articles/herringbone-artifact?lang=us. Accessed 10 Jun 2022.

24. Elster A. MRI questions. In: Spin Echo. https://mriquestions.com/spin-echo1.html

25. Mikla VI, Mikla VV. Physics of magnetic resonance imaging. In: Medical imaging technology. Elsevier; 2014. p. 39–52.

26. Delfaut EM, Beltran J, Johnson G, Rousseau J, Marchandise X, Cotten A. Fat suppression in MR imaging: techniques and pitfalls. RadioGraphics. 1999;19(2):373–82. https://doi.org/10.1148/radiographics.19.2.g99mr03373.

27. Zezo Gradient Echo. In: Radiol. Key. https://radiologykey.com/gradient-echo-part-i-basic-principles/. Accessed 10 Jun 2022.

28. Kellman P, Larson AC, Hsu L-Y, Chung Y-C, Simonetti OP, McVeigh ER, Arai AE. Motion-corrected free-breathing delayed enhancement imaging of myocardial infarction. Magn Reson Med. 2005;53(1):194–200. https://doi.org/10.1002/mrm.20333.

29. Nijm GM, Sahakian AV, Swiryn S, Carr JC, Sheehan JJ, Larson AC. Comparison of self-gated cine MRI retrospective cardiac synchronization algorithms. J Magn Reson Imaging. 2008;28(3):767–72. https://doi.org/10.1002/jmri.21514.

30. Saremi F, Grizzard JD, Kim RJ. Optimizing cardiac MR imaging: practical remedies for artifacts. RadioGraphics. 2008;28(4):1161–87. https://doi.org/10.1148/rg.284065718.

31. Alton A, Kirdar C, Özbay G. Effect of aminophylline in patients with atropine-resistant late advanced atrioventricular block during acute inferior myocardial infarction. Clin Cardiol. 1998;21(10):759–62. https://doi.org/10.1002/clc.4960211012.

32. CDC. Three things you may not know about CPR. In: CDC. 2022. https://www.cdc.gov/heart-disease/cpr.htm. Accessed 10 Jun 2022.

33. Emrich T, Emrich K, Abegunewardene N, Oberholzer K, Dueber C, Muenzel T, Kreitner K-F. Cardiac MR enables diagnosis in 90% of patients with acute chest pain, elevated bio-markers and unobstructed coronary arteries. Br J Radiol. 2015;88(1049):20150025. https://doi.org/10.1259/bjr.20150025.

Chapter 3
Ischemic Heart Disease

49. A patient is injected with gadolinium, and unfortunately 5 cc of gadolinium infiltrates into the subcutaneous tissue. The patient is asymptomatic, maintains an adequate pulse, and shows no compartmental symptoms. The management would be:

(A) Compresses and evaluation of the arm with monitoring
(B) Epinephrine
(C) Surgical consultation
(D) Opiates prescription

   The correct answer is A. Extravasation is a known complication following parenteral administration of gadolinium. Treatment included limb elevation and application of cold or warm packs [1]. Signs of anaphylaxis requiring epinephrine include wheezing, difficulty breathing, and tongue swelling, which is case report rare with gadolinium. Plastic surgeon consultation is recommended with large volume (over 50 ml) extravasation, skin ulcerations, or soft tissue necrosis sensitivity disturbances [2].

50. Which of the following is considered *inappropriate* for stress cardiac MRI?

(A) High pre-test probability of CAD (ECG uninterpretable or unable to exercise)
(B) High pre-test probability of CAD and ECG interpretable and able to exercise)
(C) Intermediate pre-test probability of CAD (ECG uninterpretable or unable to exercise)
(D) Low pre-test probability (ECG interpretable and able to exercise)

   The correct answer is D. The 2013 multi-societal guidelines have included a high pre-test probability of CAD (ECG uninterpretable or unable to exercise), high pre-test probability of CAD (ECG interpretable and able to exercise), and Intermediate pre-test probability of CAD (ECG uninterpretable or unable to exercise) as appropriate use of stress MRI. Further, for high pre-test probability of CAD (ECG uninterpretable or unable to exercise) is considered equivalent to invasive coronary angiography [3].

S. G. Al-Kindi, S. E. Janus, *Cardiac MRI Certification Exam*, https://doi.org/10.1007/978-3-031-25966-1_3

Indication Test	Exercise ECG	Stress Nuc	Stress Echo	Stress CMR	CCTA	Coronary Angiography
1 • Low Pre-Test probability of Coronary Disease • Able to Exercise and ECG interpretable	A	R	M	R	R	R
2 • Low pre-test probability of Coronary Disease • Unable to exercise or ECG Uninterpretable	X	A	A	M	M	R
3 • Intermediate pre-test probability of Coronary Disease • Able to exercise and ECG interpretable	A	A	A	M	M	R
4 • Intermediate pre-test probability of Coronary Disease • Unable to exercise or ECG uninterpretable	X	A	A	A	A	M
5 • High pre-test probability of Coronary Disease • Able to exercise and ECG interpretable	M	A	A	A	M	A
6 • High pre-test probability of Coronary Disease • Unable to exercise or ECG uninterpretable	X	A	A	A	M	A

From Wolk et al. Jacc 2013 https://www.jacc.org/doi/full/10.1016/j.jacc.2013.11.009

51. What is the most likely diagnosis?

Steady state free precession imaging   Delayed enhancement imaging

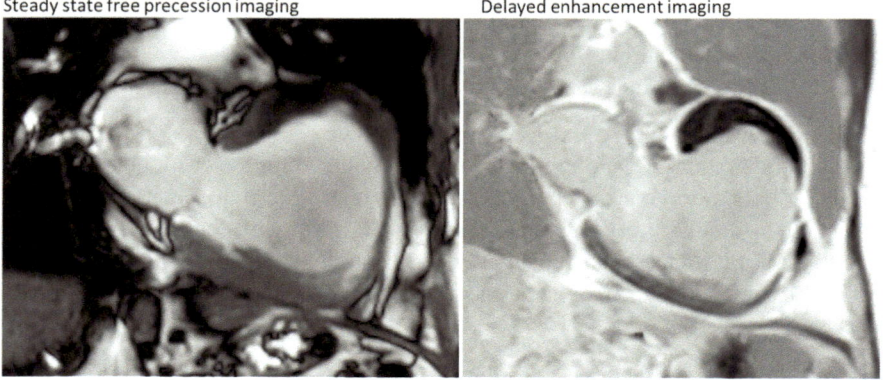

(A) Transmural apical infarction with left ventricular thrombus
(B) Transmural apical infarction without left ventricular thrombus
(C) Anterior infarction without left ventricular thrombus
(D) Anterior infarction with left ventricular thrombus

The correct answer is D. As seen in the figure below, on the two chambers (VLA—vertical long axis) there is a large transmural anterior wall infarction with aneurysm associated mural thrombus seen on the delayed imaging. If there was infarction of the apex, there would be a more distal scar and better evaluated on the four chambers (HLA—horizontal long axis) [4].

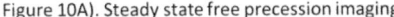

Figure 10A). Steady state free precession imaging   10B). Delayed enhancement imaging

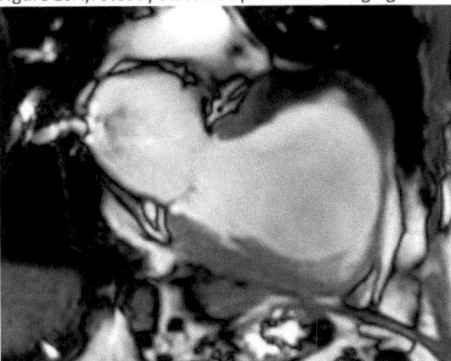 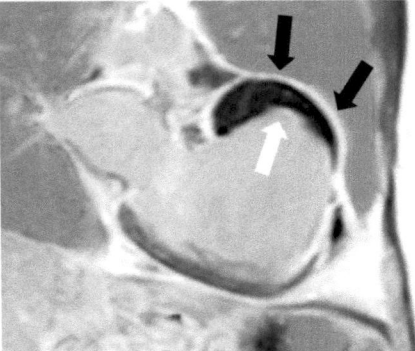

Figure 10-SSFP and delayed enhancement imaging demonstrating transmural anterior wall myocardial infarction (black arrows) with associated left ventricular mural thrombus (white arrow).

52. A 59-year-old man with a history of epilepsy arrives for a regadenoson stress MRI. After injection of regadenoson, the patient has a seizure. What is the best next step in management?

(A) Aminophylline
(B) Benzodiazepines
(C) CPR
(D) Administer gadolinium and continue imaging

The correct answer is B. When an individual experiences a seizure due to regadenoson, the recommended treatment of choice is benzodiazepines [5]. Aminophylline is not recommended as it may increase the risk of seizure and prolong the episode [6]. Gadolinium may also potentially lower the seizure threshold [7]. Bite blocks are no longer recommended in individuals with active seizures [8].

53. Which of the following would demonstrate viability based on late gadolinium imaging?

(A) 100% fibrosis
(B) 75% fibrosis
(C) 50% Fibrosis
(D) Transmural fibrosis

The correct answer is C. Any infarct comprising >50% fibrosis of the myocardial wall has a limited ability for recovery after revascularization. The correct answer is C most likely has some viability [9].

Percent fibrosis	Without Infarct	1-25%	26-50%	51-75%	>75%
Viability	Viable	Viability preserved	Viability Preserved	Viability Absent	Viability Absent
Probability of Recovery with Revascularization	80%	60%	40%	10%	2%

54. What is the most likely diagnosis on the following images?

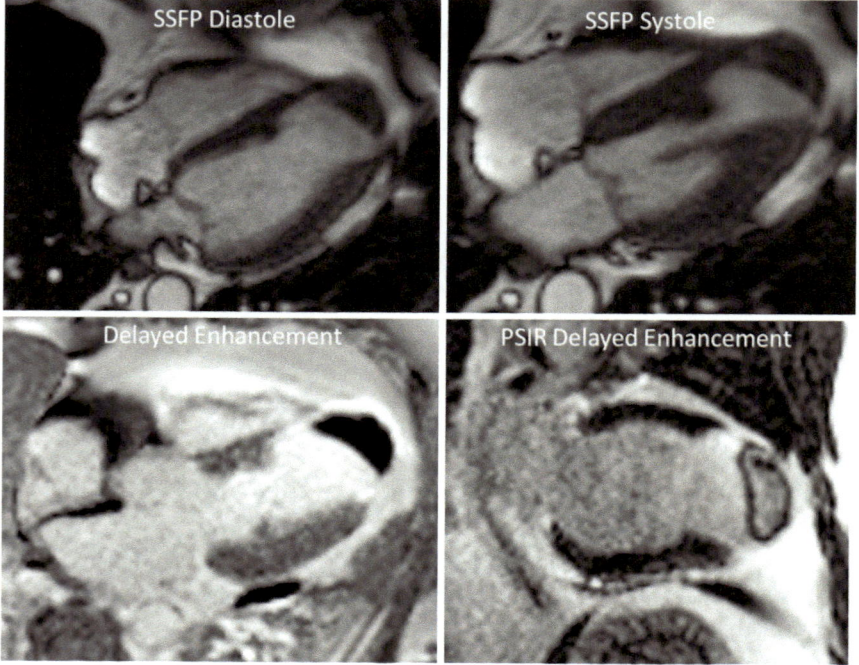

(A) LAD infarct with thrombus
(B) LAD infarct without thrombus
(C) RCA infarct with thrombus
(D) Endomyocardial fibrosis (Loeffler's syndrome)
(E) Apical hypertrophic cardiomyopathy with aneurysm and thrombus

The answer is A. The images demonstrate a large left anterior descending infarction with a mural thrombus (black arrows). The LAD infarction is transmural (white arrows) with no viability. The circumflex would be better seen in the lateral wall or short-axis lateral wall. An RCA infarct would appear in the inferior wall.

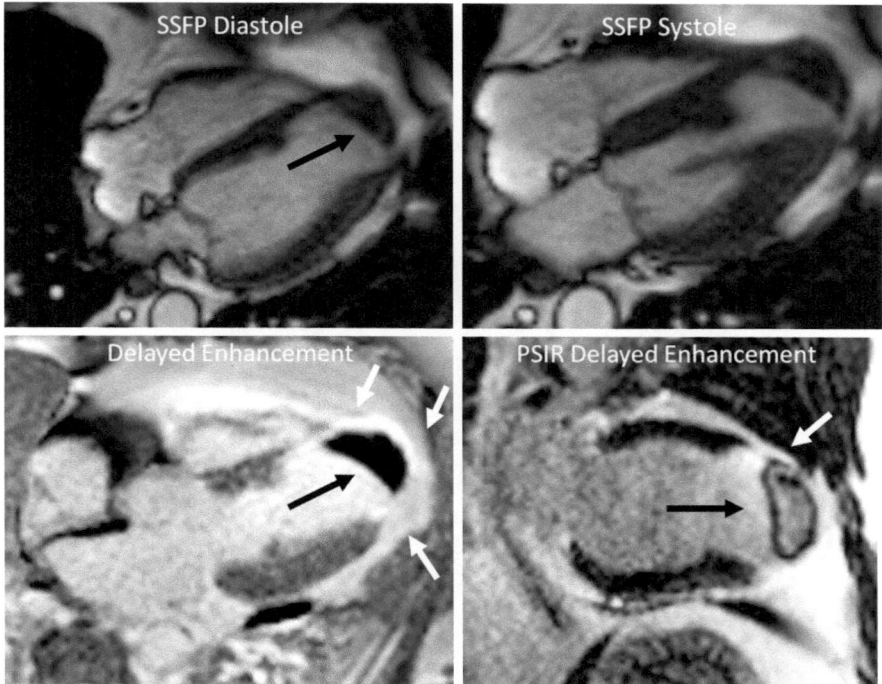

55. What is the correct interpretation of these stress images?

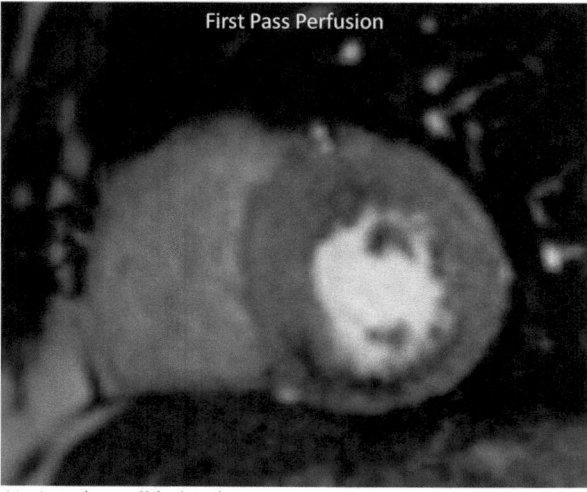

A). Anterior wall ischemia

(A) Anterior wall ischemia
(B) Inferior wall ischemia
(C) Lateral wall ischemia
(D) Septal wall ischemia
(E) Artifact

The first pass perfusion demonstrates a perfusion defect in the inferior wall demonstrating more than 1 voxel and persisting (Supplementary video Stress).

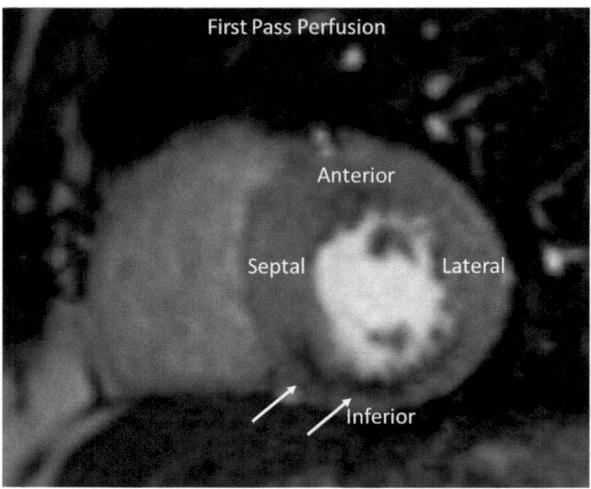

56. What is the correct interpretation of these stress images?

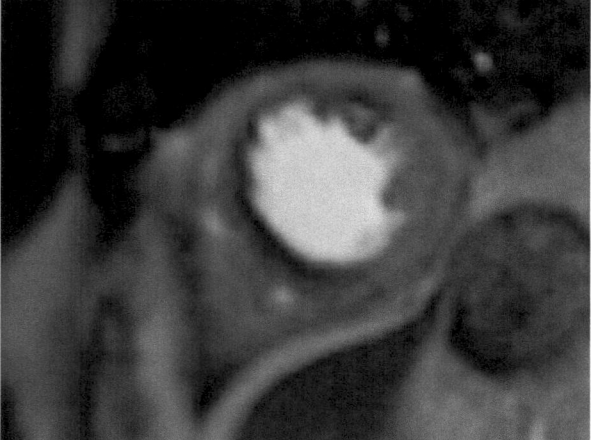

(A) Anterior wall ischemia
(B) Inferior wall ischemia

(C) Lateral wall ischemia
(D) Septal and Anterior wall ischemia
(E) Artifact

The correct answer is D. There is a moderated size territory of ischemia in the septal and anterior walls.

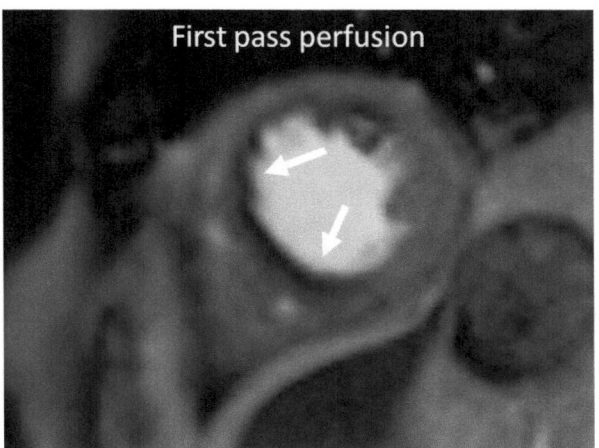

57. What is the likely diagnosis?

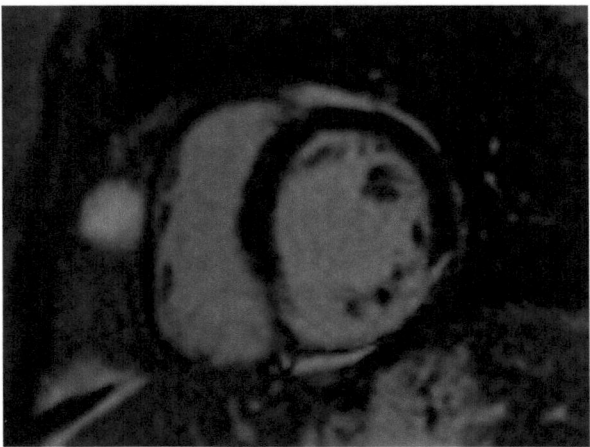

(A) Amyloid
(B) Transmural infarction
(C) Pulmonary hypertension
(D) Non-compaction

The correct answer is B. The image displays a transmural infarction in the inferior wall with no viability. Patients with pulmonary hypertension often have RV insertion site fibrosis and dilated RV, which is not seen here. There is no evidence of non-compaction, which would show significant trabeculation. Amyloid is more of a diffuse fibrosis process, while this follows a certain coronary territory making ischemia much more likely.

58. What is the most likely diagnosis?

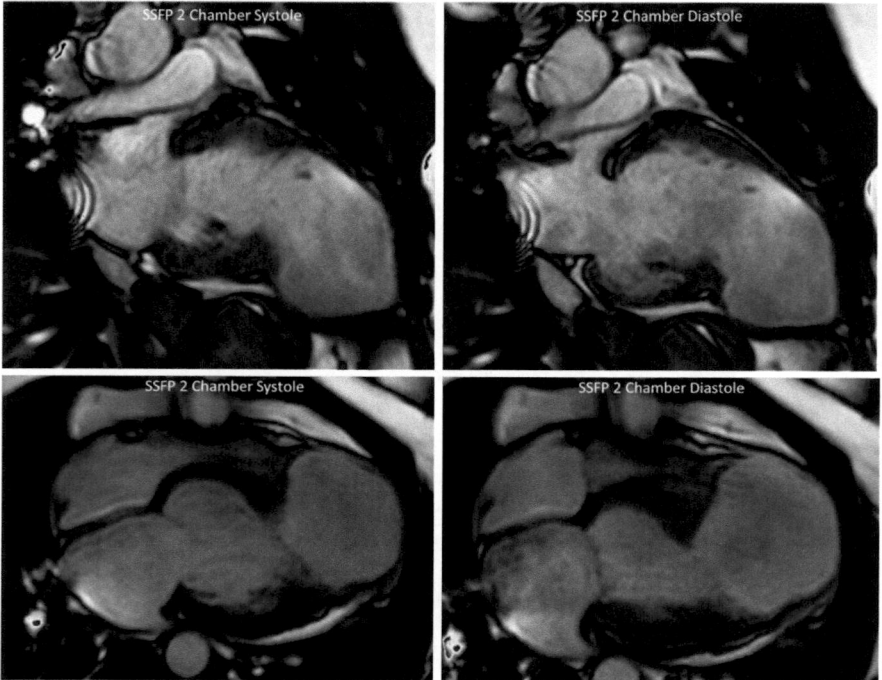

(A) LV apical aneurysm
(B) LV pseudoaneurysm
(C) Takotsubo cardiomyopathy
(D) Apical Hypertrophic cardiomyopathy

The correct answer is B. The images demonstrate a large pseudoaneurysm [10]. LV pseudoaneurysm develops when there is myocardial contained rupture and there only remains pericardium without myocardium as the border. These images demonstrate a narrow neck, which is common in an LV pseudoaneurysm. While Takotsubo cardiomyopathy demonstrates apical ballooning, it should still have myocardium within the walls. An apical aneurysm usually demonstrates a wide neck, not a narrow neck and maintains myocardium in the borders. Apical hypertrophic cardiomyopathy would have left ventricular hypertrophy, not thinning.

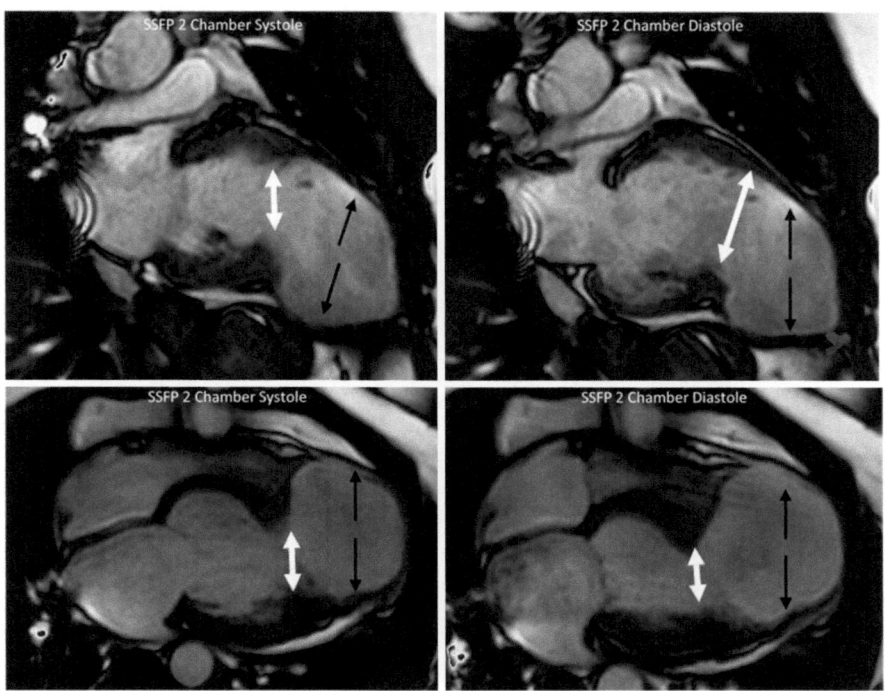

White arrows demonstrating narrow neck of LV pseudo aneurysm. The black arrows indicate the absence of myocardium at the wall/borders.

59. What is the most likely diagnosis based on the image below?

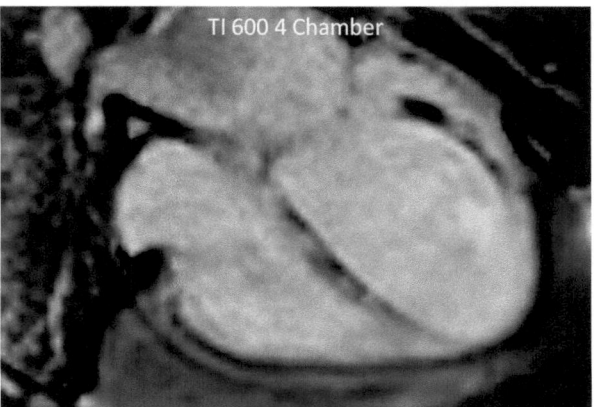

(A) Multiple mural thrombi
(B) Microvascular obstruction
(C) Myocarditis
(D) Clot in transit

   The correct answer is B. The image is a TI600 demonstrating microvascular obstruction in the septal and lateral walls [11].

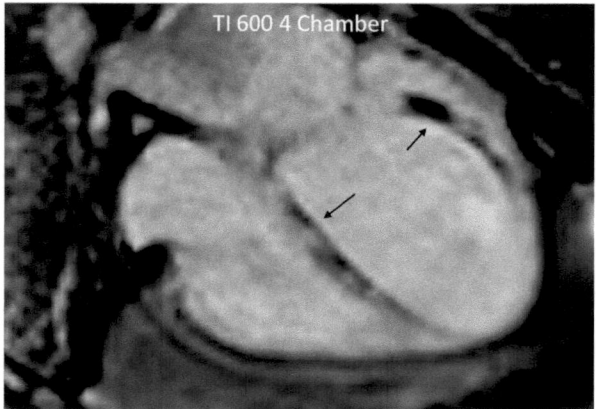

Black arrows demonstrating areas of microvascular dysfunction.

60. What is the likely diagnosis?

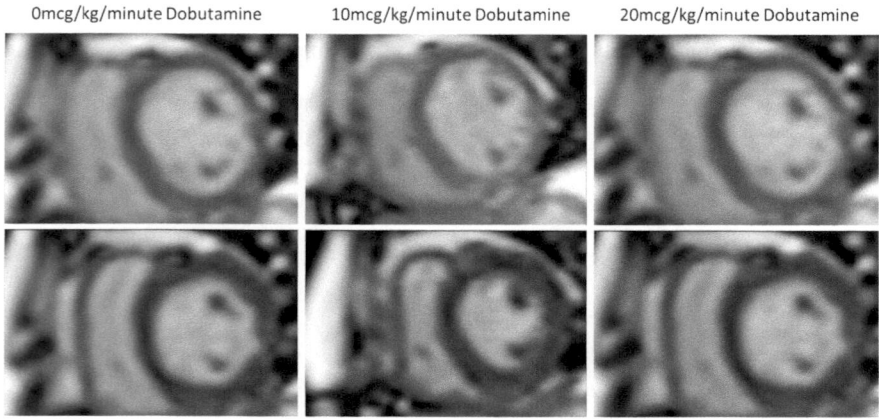

(A) Infarct
(B) Ischemia
(C) Scared
(D) Normal

The correct answer is B. The images demonstrate a biphasic response to dobutamine. There is improved systolic function at the 10 mcg dose, however, the function then declines at the 20-mcg dose. This is seen typically with ischemia or ischemic/viable myocardium. Scared myocardium would not improve, neither would infarcted myocardium. Normal myocardium would continue to improve at a 20-mcg dose which is not seen here. See supplemental videos.

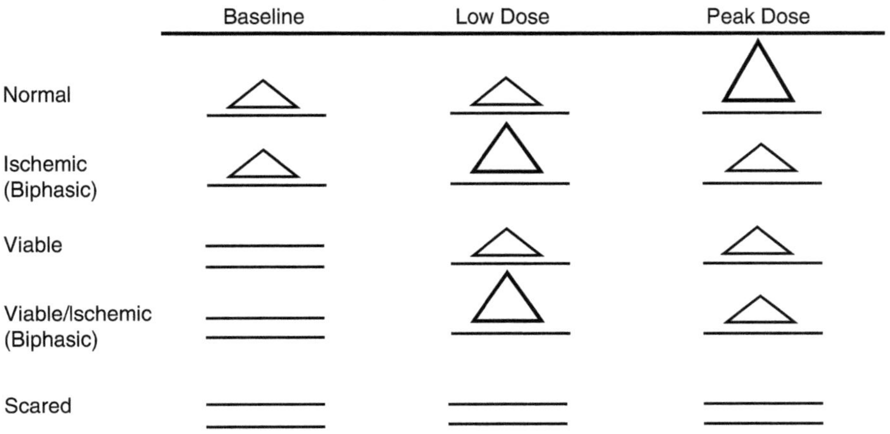

	Baseline	Low Dose	Peak Dose
Normal	△	△	△
Ischemic (Biphasic)	△	△	△
Viable		△	△
Viable/Ischemic (Biphasic)		△	△
Scared			

61. Which of the following is an incorrect strategy to use for patients with mis-triggering arrhythmias?

(A) Reapply new ECG pads
(B) Use navigator gating (liver dome)
(C) Alter which leads you gate/trigger from
(D) Remove chest hair prior to applying ECG pads

The correct answer is B. Triggering still requires cardiac gating with ECG. Navigator gating is used for respiratory gating in 3D imaging. Reapplying new ECG pads, removing excessive hair, or changing which lead you trigger from are all correct strategies to deal with mis-triggering arrhythmias.

62. What is the most likely diagnosis?

WB MOCO FLASH PSIR

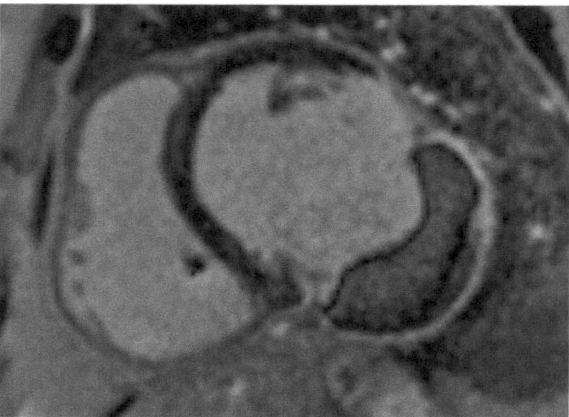

(A) LAD infarct
(B) Circumflex infarct
(C) Circumflex infarct with microvascular obstruction
(D) Pseudoaneurysm with mural thrombus

The correct answer is D. While B is partially correct in that there is a Left circumflex infarct. The most striking finding part of the image is the large thrombus and pseudoaneurysm located in the lateral-infero-lateral wall. There is no enhancement in the anterior wall to suggest LAD infarction. There is no evidence of microvascular obstruction.

WB MOCO FLASH PSIR

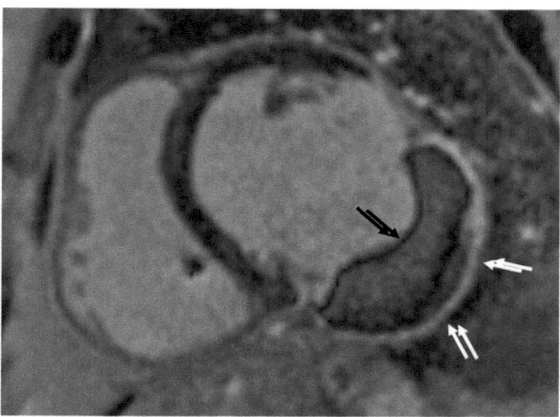

WB MOCO FLASH PSIR- demonstrating pseudoaneurysm (white arrow) in the basal lateral-inferior wall with large thrombus burden (black arrow)

References

1. Bellin M-F, Jakobsen JÅ, Tomassin I, Thomsen HS, Morcos SK, members of the *Contrast Media Safe. Contrast medium extravasation injury: guidelines for prevention and management. Eur Radiol. 2002;12(11):2807–12. https://doi.org/10.1007/s00330-002-1630-9.
2. Tonolini M. Extravasation of gadolinium-based contrast medium. In: Eurorad. https://www.eurorad.org/case/9405. Accessed 10 Jun 2022.
3. Wolk MJ, Bailey SR, Doherty JU, Douglas PS, Hendel RC, Kramer CM, Min JK, Patel MR, Rosenbaum L, Shaw LJ, Stainback RF, Allen JM. ACCF/AHA/ASE/ASNC/HFSA/HRS/SCAI/SCCT/SCMR/STS 2013 Multimodality Appropriate Use Criteria for the Detection and Risk Assessment of Stable Ischemic Heart Disease. J Am Coll Cardiol. 2014;63(4):380–406. https://doi.org/10.1016/j.jacc.2013.11.009.
4. Pöss J, Desch S, Eitel C, de Waha S, Thiele H, Eitel I. Left ventricular thrombus formation after ST-segment–elevation myocardial infarction: insights from a cardiac magnetic resonance multicenter study. Circ Cardiovasc Imaging. 2015;8(10):e003417. https://doi.org/10.1161/CIRCIMAGING.115.003417.
5. Andrikopoulou E, Hage FG. Adverse effects associated with regadenoson myocardial perfusion imaging. J Nucl Cardiol. 2018;25(5):1724–31. https://doi.org/10.1007/s12350-018-1218-7.
6. Astellas Lexiscan Indications and Important Safety Information. In: Lexiscan Indic. Important Saf. Inf. https://lexiscan.com/ClinicalAttributes/Overview#:~:text=New%2Donset%20or%20recurrence%20of,seizures%20associated%20with%20Lexiscan%20injection. Accessed 28 Aug 2022.
7. Gordin V. Gadolinium encephalopathy after intrathecal gadolinium injection. Pain Physician. 2010;13(5):E321–6. https://doi.org/10.36076/ppj.2010/13/E321.
8. Billington M, Kandalaft O, Aisiku I. Adult status epilepticus: a review of the prehospital and emergency department management. J Clin Med. 2016;5(9):74. https://doi.org/10.3390/jcm5090074.
9. Souto ALM, Souto RM, Teixeira ICR, Nacif MS. Myocardial viability on cardiac magnetic resonance. Arq Bras Cardiol. 2017. https://doi.org/10.5935/abc.20170056
10. Mousavi N, Buksak R, Walker JR, Hussain F, Pascoe E, Kirkpatrick IDC, Jassal DS. Left ventricular pseudoaneurysm: the role of multimodality cardiac imaging. Can J Cardiol. 2009;25(11):e389. https://doi.org/10.1016/S0828-282X(09)70168-0.
11. Sahu A. CMR imaging of profound macrovascular obstruction; 8.

Chapter 4
Nonischemic Heart Disease

63. What is the most likely diagnosis in the following images?

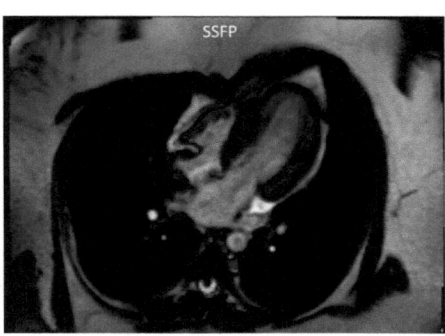 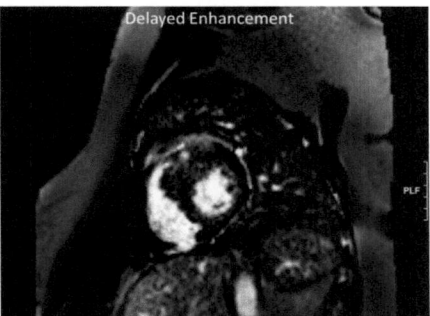

(A) Hypertrophic cardiomyopathy
(B) Sarcoidosis
(C) Myocardial infarction
(D) Arrhythmogenic right ventricular dysplasia

The correct answer is A. There is significant septal hypertrophy and scaring seen on delayed imaging. Sarcoidosis would normally involve a patchy distribution of delayed enhancement. Myocardial infarction will demonstrate a coronary territory [1]. Arrhythmogenic dysplasia would involve scaring or fatty infiltration of the right ventricle.

S. G. Al-Kindi, S. E. Janus, *Cardiac MRI Certification Exam*, https://doi.org/10.1007/978-3-031-25966-1_4

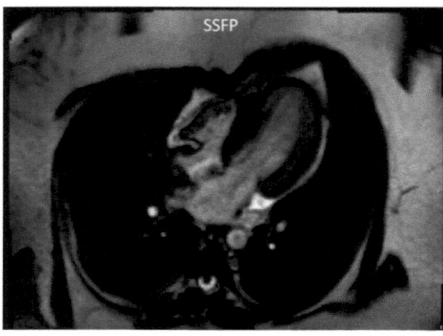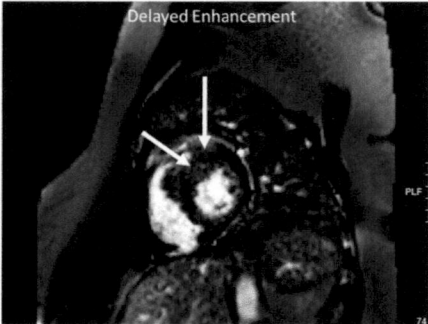

64. What is the most likely diagnosis?

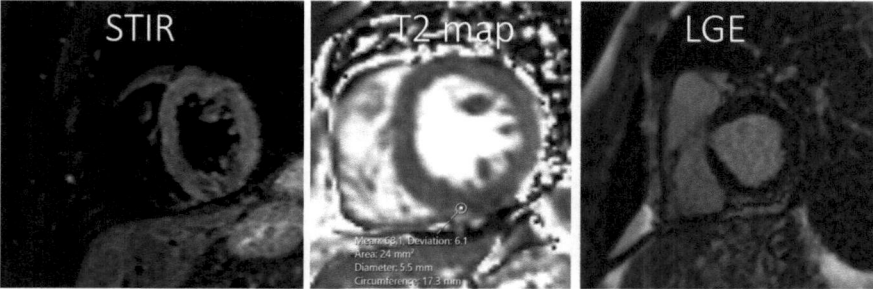

(A) Sarcoidosis
(B) Transmural infarct
(C) Viral myocarditis
(D) Pericarditis

The correct answer is C. The T2 imaging showing the HLA (horizontal long axis) of the heart demonstrates elevation (>55 msec) in the mid-lateral wall [2]. This is a common spot (mid-inferolateral) wall spot that myocarditis normally involves. Sarcoidosis presents as more a patchy fibrosis with multiple spots of involvement, but can involve the mid-inferolateral wall [3]. Pericarditis would involve enhancement of the pericardium on Short tau inversion recovery (STIR) or delayed enhancement imaging.

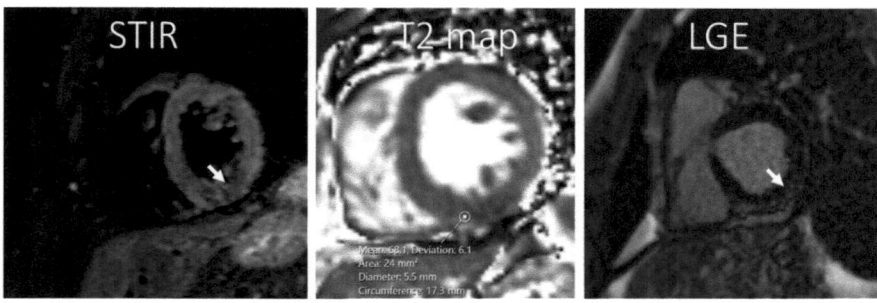

65. What is the most likely diagnosis?

T1 Map

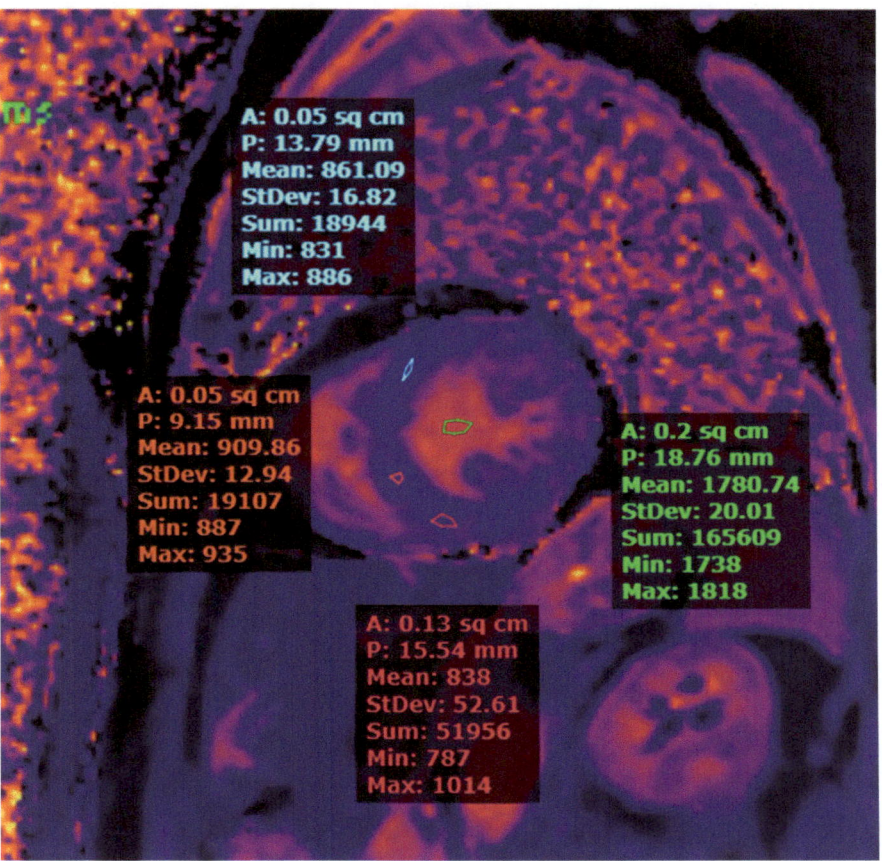

(A) Fabry's disease
(B) Myocarditis
(C) Infarction
(D) Sarcoidosis

The correct answer is A, Fabry's disease. The T1 series demonstrates abnormally low T1 values which are indicative of fatty infiltration of the myocardium [4]. Myocarditis, infarction, and sarcoidosis would result in elevated T1 values due to disruption of cell membranes [5].

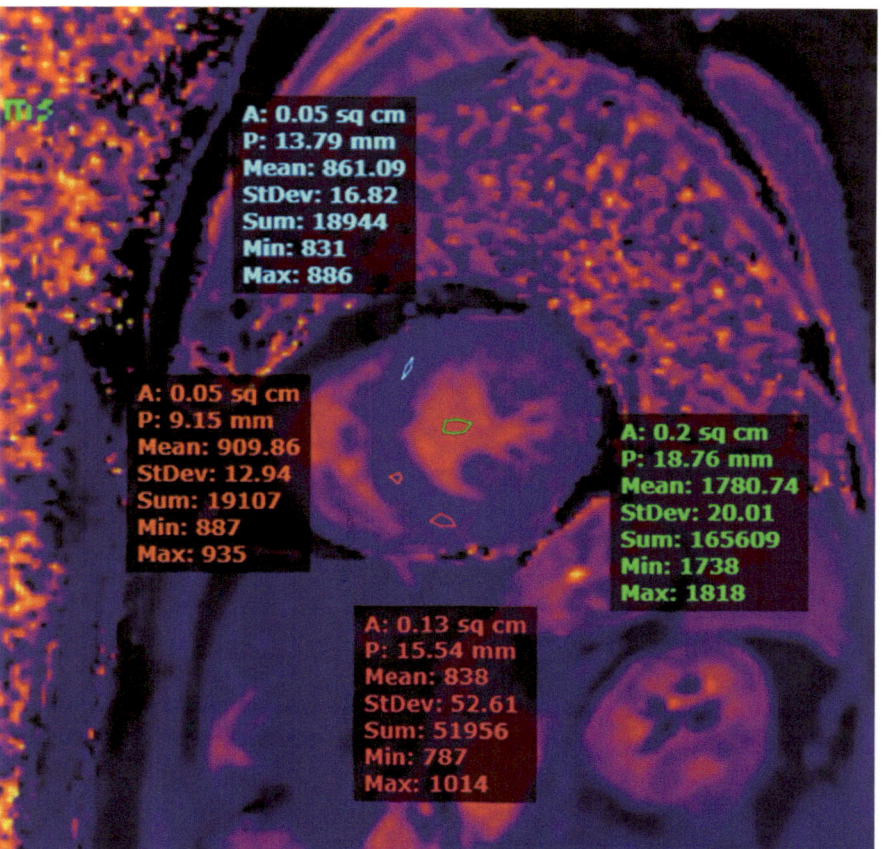

T1 Map demonstrating abnormally low
myocardial values representative of fatty
infiltration which can be seen in Fabry's
disease.

66. What is the most likely diagnosis on this T2* series?

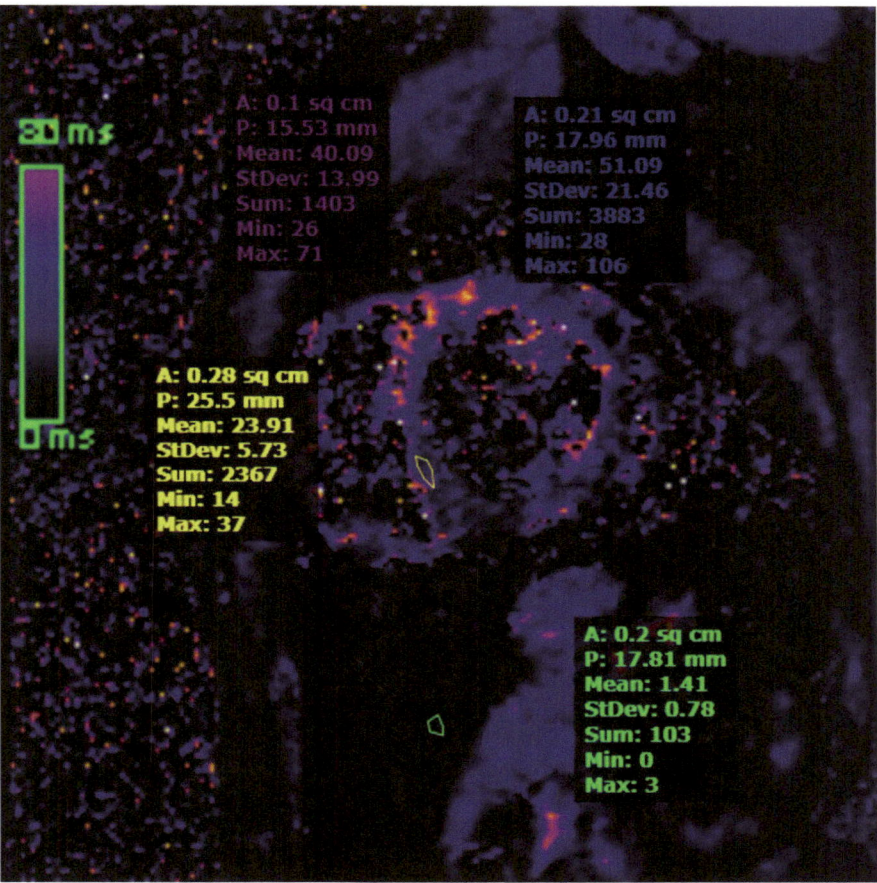

(A) Hepatic Iron overload
(B) Hepatic and Myocardial iron overload
(C) Myocardial overload
(D) Neither hepatic nor myocardial iron overload

The correct answer is A. On this T2*series, there is hepatic iron overload with T2* value of 1.41 msec, meanwhile, there is relatively normal myocardium with T2* values of 23–51 msec [6]. Myocardial T2* values <20 ms represent accumulation of iron. One can easily see the dark texture of the liver compared to the relatively normal myocardium.

67. The following images likely represent a diagnosis of?

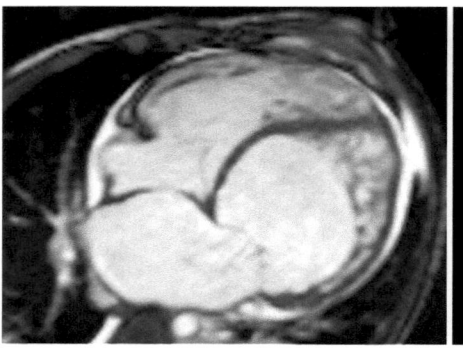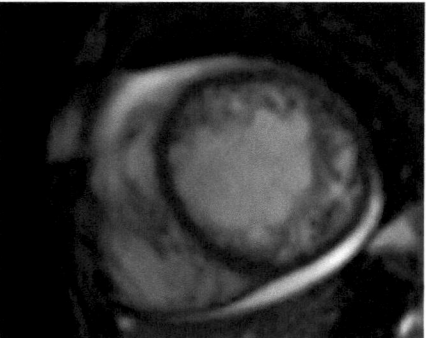

(A) Idiopathic dilated cardiomyopathy
(B) Ischemic cardiomyopathy
(C) Arrhythmogenic right ventricular dysplasia
(D) Non-compaction cardiomyopathy

The correct answer is D. Left ventricular non-compaction is the most likely answer. Based on the Peterson criteria in the four chambers the non-compacted to compacted myocardium measures >2.3. Additionally, on the short axis the Stacey criteria show a non-compacted to compacted ratio >2. The images also show evidence of RV non-compaction (which is less well characterized). This does not appear to be a case of idiopathic cardiomyopathy as there is substantial non-compacted myocardium. While the right ventricle is dilated, it also demonstrates significant non-compacted myocardium which is not consistent with ARVC. There is no evidence of ischemia as the cause of the dilated left ventricular size.

68. What is the most common delayed enhancement pattern in idiopathic dilated cardiomyopathies?

(A) Sub-endocardial apical
(B) Inferior wall mid-myocardial
(C) Mid-myocardial septal wall
(D) Septal sub-endomyocardial

The correct answer is C. The most common enhancement pattern in dilated cardiomyopathy is mid-wall in the basal septum of the left ventricle [7]. Sub-endomyocardial fibrosis typically involves infarct/ischemia. Mid-myocardial in the inferior-lateral area is typically associated with myocarditis or sarcoidosis.

Delayed Enhancement Imaging

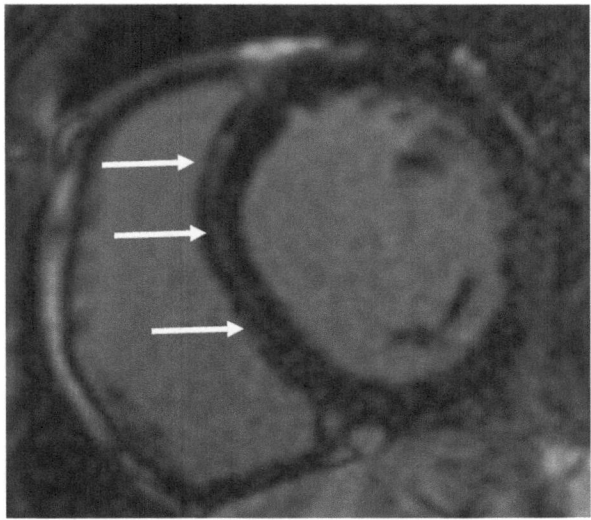

69. What is the most likely diagnosis based on the images below?

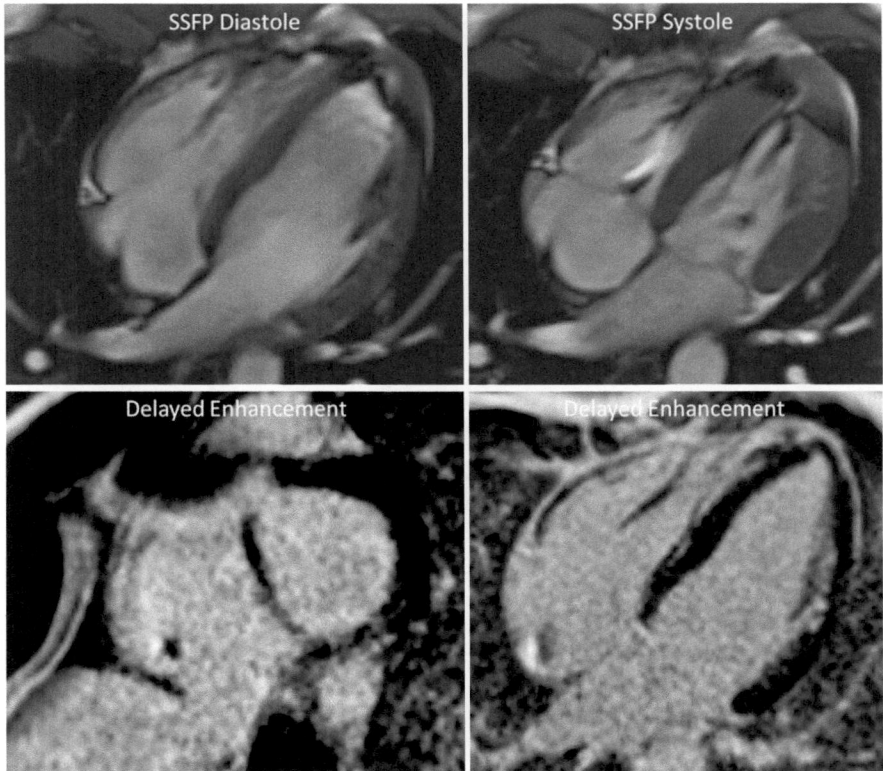

(A) Ischemic cardiomyopathy
(B) Sarcoidosis
(C) Arrhythmogenic right ventricular dysplasia
(D) Myocarditis

The correct answer is C. As seen in the images, the RV is dilated and there is focal fibrosis in the right ventricular basal segment and in the right ventricular septum. There is preserved contraction in the apex of the right ventricle, however, the base demonstrates hypertrophy and dyskinesia (supplemental video), making the diagnosis likely Arrhythmogenic right ventricular dysplasia [8]. There is no evidence of patchy fibrosis to suggest sarcoidosis. There is no mid-myocardial fibrosis to suggest myocarditis. There is no sub-endomyocardial enhancement to suggest ischemic territory.

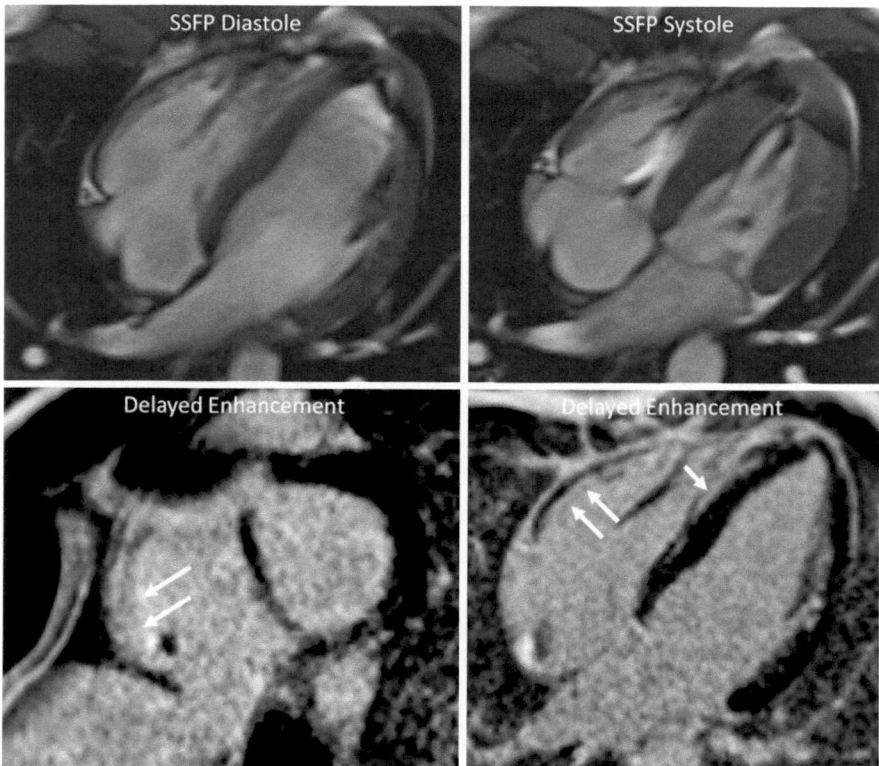

70. What is the most likely diagnosis below?

Delayed Enhancement

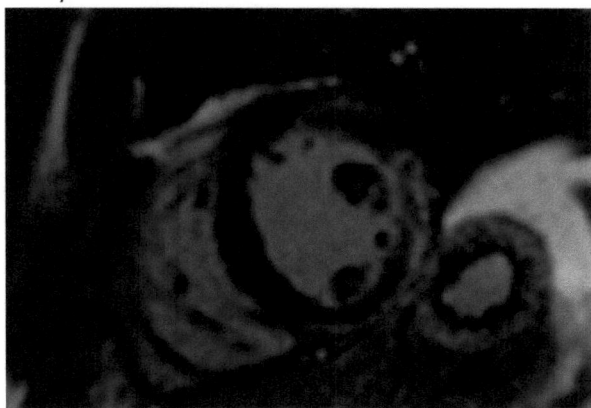

(A) Myocarditis
(B) Sub-endomyocardial infarction
(C) Transmural myocardial infarction
(D) Idiopathic dilated cardiomyopathy

The correct answer is A. The image demonstrates a significant mid-myocardial scar in the inferior-lateral enhancement making myocarditis the correct choice [9]. There is no evidence of transmural myocardial or sub-endomyocardial infarction. There is significant scaring in the lateral wall, which argues against idiopathic cardiomyopathy.

Delayed Enhancement

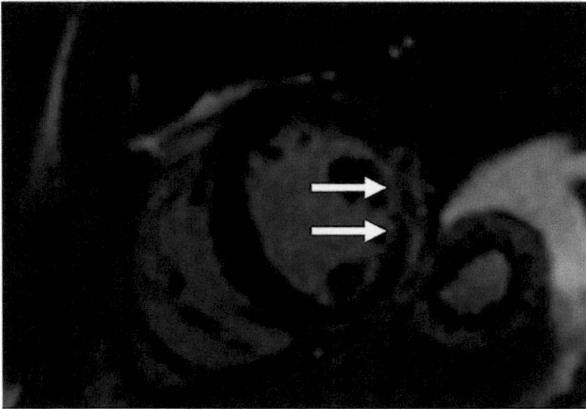

Delayed Enhancement – demonstrating significant mid myocardial scar in the lateral and inferio-lateral wall (white arrow)

71. What is demonstrated in the following images?

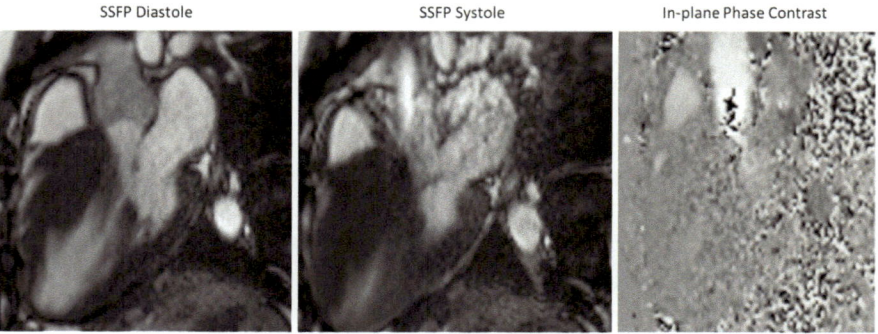

(A) Aortic regurgitation
(B) Mitral stenosis
(C) Amyloid
(D) Systolic anterior motion

The correct answer is D. The in-plane imaging demonstrates dephasing in the outflow tract during systole from systolic anterior motion of the mitral valve from the venturi effect due to left ventricular hypertrophy [10]. This is a likely case of hypertrophic cardiomyopathy. Amyloid sometimes can present with systolic anterior motion and LV hypertrophy, but is less likely than hypertrophic cardiomyopathy, and would require late gadolinium imaging for confirmation. While aortic insufficiency can result in increased systolic velocities, the asymmetric LV hypertrophy and systolic anterior motion are not characteristic.

72. A 18-year-old male with a past medical history of COVID-19 presents with chest pain. High sensitivity troponin 200 pg/dL, sed rate 56, CRP 12, with echo demonstrating EF of 40%. CTA coronaries demonstrate normal coronary arteries. Primary team requests a cardiac MRI. What is the most likely diagnosis based on the images?

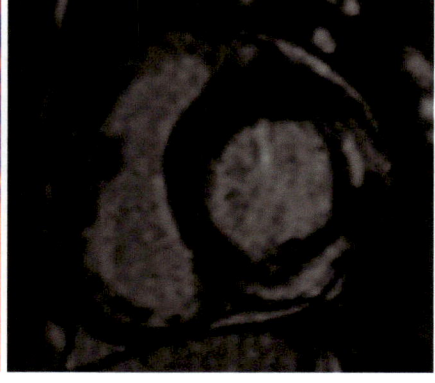

(A) Myocarditis
(B) Kawasaki with LAD aneurysm
(C) Cocaine-induced vasospasm
(D) Sarcoidosis
(E) Takotsubo cardiomyopathy

The correct answer is A. The T2 map demonstrates an elevated area of signal in the mid-myocardium of the basal inferior and basal lateral walls of myocarditis [9]. These are typical locations of myocardial inflammation/myocarditis. The late gadolinium imaging demonstrates enhancement in the same areas. This does not represent fibrosis but just membrane disruption of the cell membranes. There is no evidence of LAD aneurysm, especially with a normal CT coronary angiogram. There was no hint of involvement of cocaine-induced vasospasm. Takotsubo would give apical ballooning typically seen in the four chamber. Sarcoidosis can affect the basal inferior and basal lateral wall, but typically gives a more patchy appearance and has conduction abnormalities or lung findings in addition.

73. A 48-year-old female with a past medical history of Mobitz II heart block s/p loop recorder was referred to MRI for a workup of cardiomyopathy. The most likely diagnosis based on the images is?

T2 Map   Late Gadolinium Imaging

(A) Sarcoidosis
(B) Myocarditis
(C) Infarction
(D) ARVC

The correct answer is A Sarcoidosis [3]. The T2 map demonstrates significant elevation in T2 signal corresponding to active edema in the septum where the AV node and bundle branches run. The late gadolinium enhancement in the septum shows cell membrane disruption. Given the clinical scenario of heart block, sarcoidosis should be high on the differential. Myocarditis would present with viral symptoms. ARVC would have hypertrophy or dyskinesia in the right ventricle. There is no evidence of infarction or sub-endomyocardial infarction.

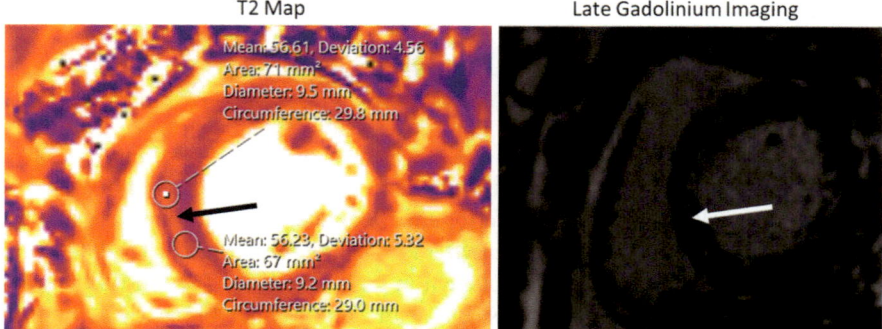

T2 Map- demonstrating area of high signal (black arrow, >55msec) indicating edema or inflammation. Late gadolinium enhancement demonstrating area of enhancement (cell membrane disruption, white arrow).

74. What is the most likely diagnosis?

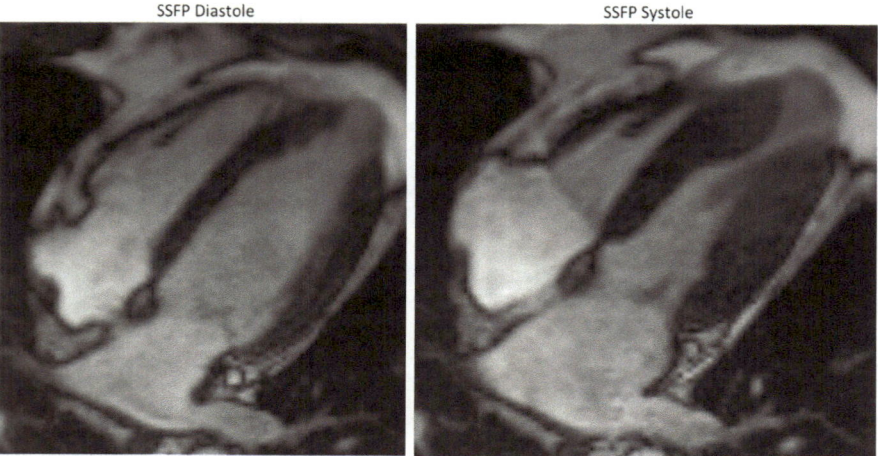

(A) Myocarditis
(B) ARVC
(C) Yamaguchi syndrome
(D) Eosinophilic myocarditis

The correct answer is Yamaguchi syndrome or apical hypertrophic cardiomyopathy [11]. The images demonstrate apical LV hypertrophy with an apical aneurysm. ARVC would show some dyskinesia in the right ventricle.

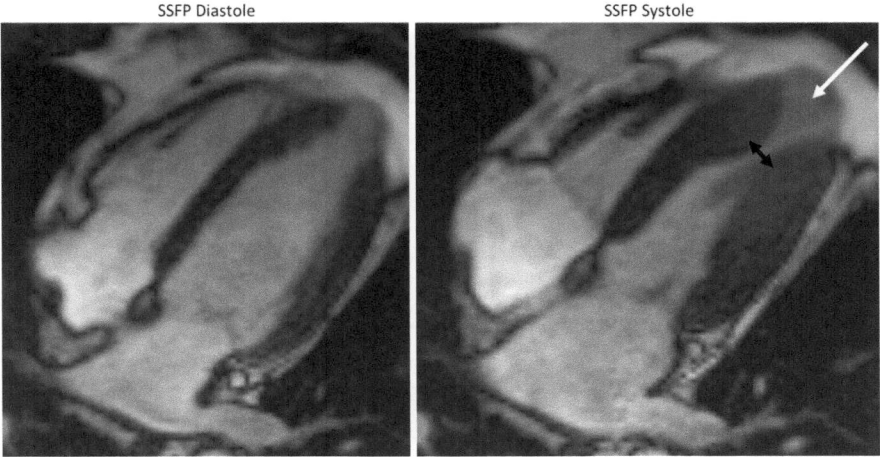

75. What is the most likely diagnosis?

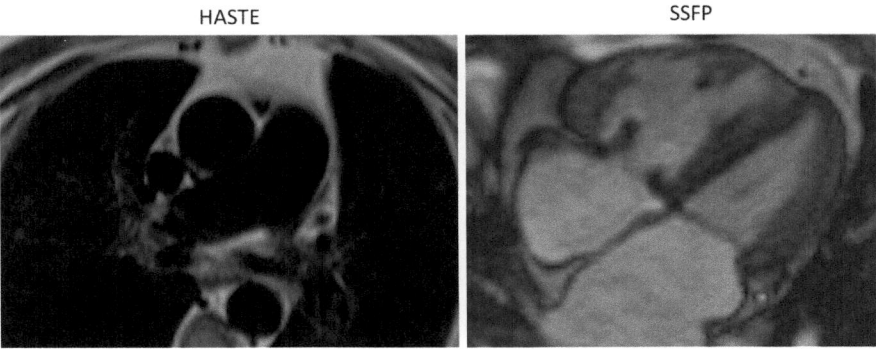

(A) Pulmonary hypertension with right ventricular hypertrophy/failure
(B) Pulmonary hypertension with normal right ventricular function
(C) Arrhythmogenic right ventricular dysplasia
(D) Myocarditis

The correct answer is pulmonary hypertension with right ventricular failure. The pulmonary artery is dilated in the HASTE images. Pulmonary artery greater than 3 cm, indicates likely pulmonary hypertension. The images of the right ventricle demonstrate severe dilation and dysfunction seen with end-stage pulmonary hypertension [12]. Arrhythmogenic right ventricular dysplasia would not cause dilation of the main pulmonary artery. Myocarditis can affect the right ventricle, but should not affect the pulmonary artery.

HASTE   SSFP

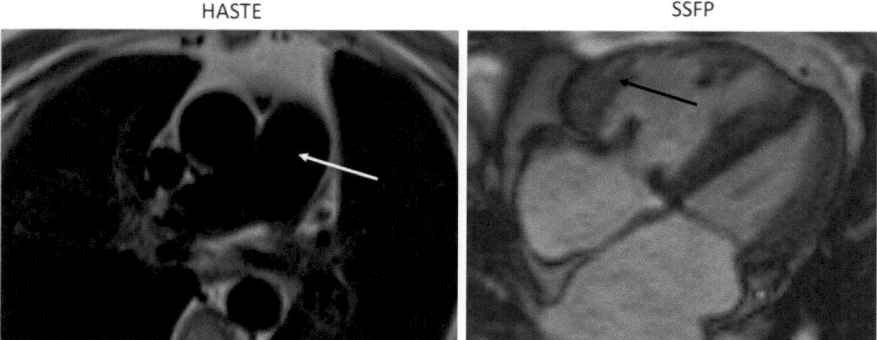

HASTE imaging demonstrating severely dilated pulmonary artery (white arrow) greater than 3cm, which indicates pulmonary hypertension. SSFP demonstrating right ventricular enlargement (black arrow) and D shaped septum which indicates RV volume/pressure overload.

76. What is the most likely diagnosis based on the images below?

Delayed Enhancement

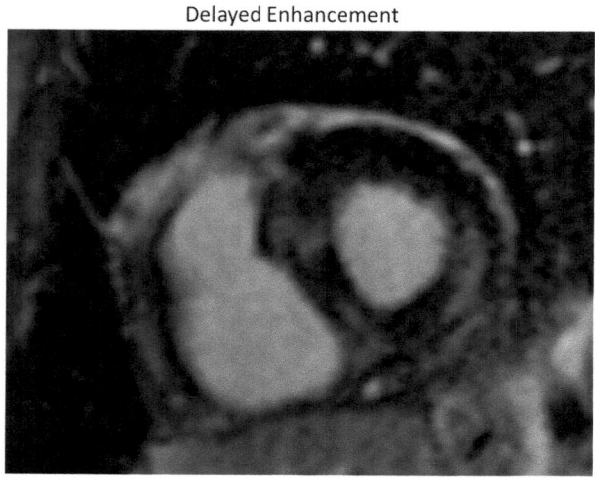

(A) Amyloid
(B) Myocarditis
(C) LAD infarction
(D) RCA infarction

The correct answer is A. The images demonstrate hypertrophied ventricle with diffuse fibrosis. The pattern of increased basal fibrosis and mid-myocardial and sub-endomyocardial fibrosis is consistent with a diagnosis of amyloid [13]. Myocarditis would have only a mid-myocardial pattern. LAD and RCA infarctions would stay within their coronary territories of the anterior and inferior walls, respectively.

Delayed Enhancement

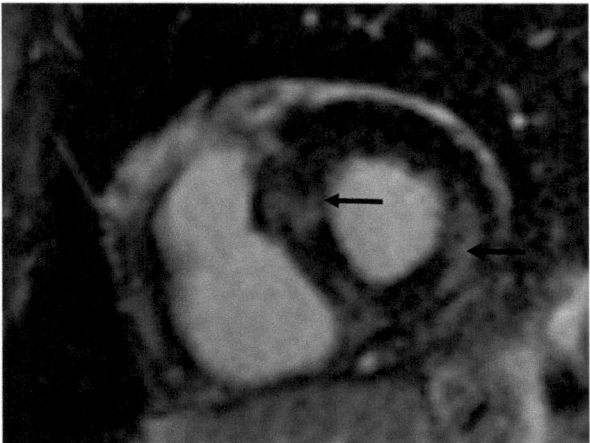

Delayed Enhancement- demonstrating
multiple areas of mid myocardial fibrosis
(black arrows) in a hypertrophied small
ventricle

77. Which of the following is not a major criterion in the 2010 ARVC Task force
criteria for ARVC?

(A) Regional RV contraction abnormality
(B) RVEDVI ≥ 110 ml/m² for men
(C) RVEDVI ≥ 90 ml/m² in women
(D) Global RV dysfunction ≤40%

The correct answer is C. The major criteria for ARVC are regional RV contraction abnormality (akinesia/dyskinesia/dyssynchrony) along with RV enlargement (Major RVEDVI ≥110 ml/m² for men, ≥100 ml/m² for women) and/or global RV dysfunction major RVEF ≤40%. RVEDVI >90 ml/m² is a minor criterion for women as is RVEDVI ≥100 ml/m² for men). To fulfill the overall criteria for ARVC definitive you need 2 major or 1 major and 2 minor criteria (global or regional dysfunction, tissue characterization of wall via endomyocardial biopsy, repolarization abnormalities, and depolarization abnormalities on ECG, arrhythmias on CG or family history) [14].

References

1. Amano Y, Kitamura M, Takano H, Yanagisawa F, Tachi M, Suzuki Y, Kumita S, Takayama M. Cardiac MR imaging of hypertrophic cardiomyopathy: techniques, findings, and clinical relevance. Magn Reson Med Sci. 2018;17(2):120–31. https://doi.org/10.2463/mrms.rev.2017-0145.
2. Sechtem U, Mahrholdt H, Vogelsberg H. Cardiac magnetic resonance in myocardial disease. Heart. 2006;93(12):1520–7. https://doi.org/10.1136/hrt.2005.067355.
3. Hulten E, Aslam S, Osborne M, Abbasi S, Bittencourt MS. Cardiac sarcoidosis—state of the art review. Cardiovasc Diagn Ther. 2016;6(1):14.
4. Germain P, Ghannudi SE, Jeung M-Y, Ohlmann P, Epailly E, Roy C, Gangi A. Native T1 mapping of the heart – a pictorial review. Clin Med Insights Cardiol. 2014;8s4:CMC.S19005. https://doi.org/10.4137/CMC.S19005
5. Mavrogeni S, Apostolou D, Argyriou P, Velitsista S, Papa L, Efentakis S, Vernardos E, Kanoupaki M, Kanoupakis G, Manginas A. T1 and T2 mapping in cardiology: "mapping the obscure object of desire". Cardiology. 2017;138(4):207–17. https://doi.org/10.1159/000478901.
6. Taghizadeh Sarvestani R, Moradveisi B, Kompany F, Ghaderi E. Correlation between heart and liver iron levels measured by MRI T2* and serum ferritin in patients with β-thalassemia Major. Int J Pediatr. 2016;4(3) https://doi.org/10.22038/ijp.2016.6587.
7. Franco A, Javidi S, Ruehm SG. Delayed myocardial enhancement in cardiac magnetic resonance imaging. J Radiol Case Rep. 2015;9(6):6–18. https://doi.org/10.3941/jrcr.v9i6.2328.
8. Tavano A, Maurel B, Gaubert J-Y, Varoquaux A, Cassagneau P, Vidal V, Bartoli J-M, Moulin G, Jacquier A. MR imaging of arrhythmogenic right ventricular dysplasia: what the radiologist needs to know. Diagn Interv Imaging. 2015;96(5):449–60. https://doi.org/10.1016/j.diii.2014.07.009.
9. Friedrich MG, Marcotte F. Cardiac magnetic resonance assessment of myocarditis. Circ Cardiovasc Imaging. 2013;6(5):833–9. https://doi.org/10.1161/CIRCIMAGING.113.000416.
10. Medical Masterclass contributors, Firth J. Cardiology: hypertrophic cardiomyopathy. Clin Med. 2019;19(1):61–3. https://doi.org/10.7861/clinmedicine.19-1-61.
11. Kennedy A, Hu RA. Case of Yamaguchi syndrome – a rare variant of hypertrophic. Cardiomyopathy 3.
12. Raymond TE, Khabbaza JE, Yadav R, Tonelli AR. Significance of main pulmonary artery dilation on imaging studies. Ann Am Thorac Soc. 2014;11(10):1623–32. https://doi.org/10.1513/AnnalsATS.201406-253PP.
13. Pucci A, Aimo A, Musetti V, Barison A, Vergaro G, Genovesi D, Giorgetti A, Masotti S, Arzilli C, Prontera C, Pastormerlo LE, Coceani MA, Ciardetti M, Martini N, Palmieri C, Passino C, Rapezzi C, Emdin M. Amyloid deposits and fibrosis on left ventricular endomyocardial biopsy correlate with extracellular volume in cardiac amyloidosis. J Am Heart Assoc. 2021;10(20):e020358. https://doi.org/10.1161/JAHA.120.020358.
14. Pieles GE, Grosse-Wortmann L, Hader M, Fatah M, Chungsomprasong P, Slorach C, Hui W, Fan C-PS, Manlhiot C, Mertens L, Hamilton R, Friedberg MK. Association of echocardiographic parameters of right ventricular remodeling and myocardial performance with modified task force criteria in adolescents with arrhythmogenic right ventricular cardiomyopathy. Circ Cardiovasc Imaging. 2019;12(4):e007693. https://doi.org/10.1161/CIRCIMAGING.118.007693.

Chapter 5
Pericardial Disease

78. What is the most likely diagnosis?

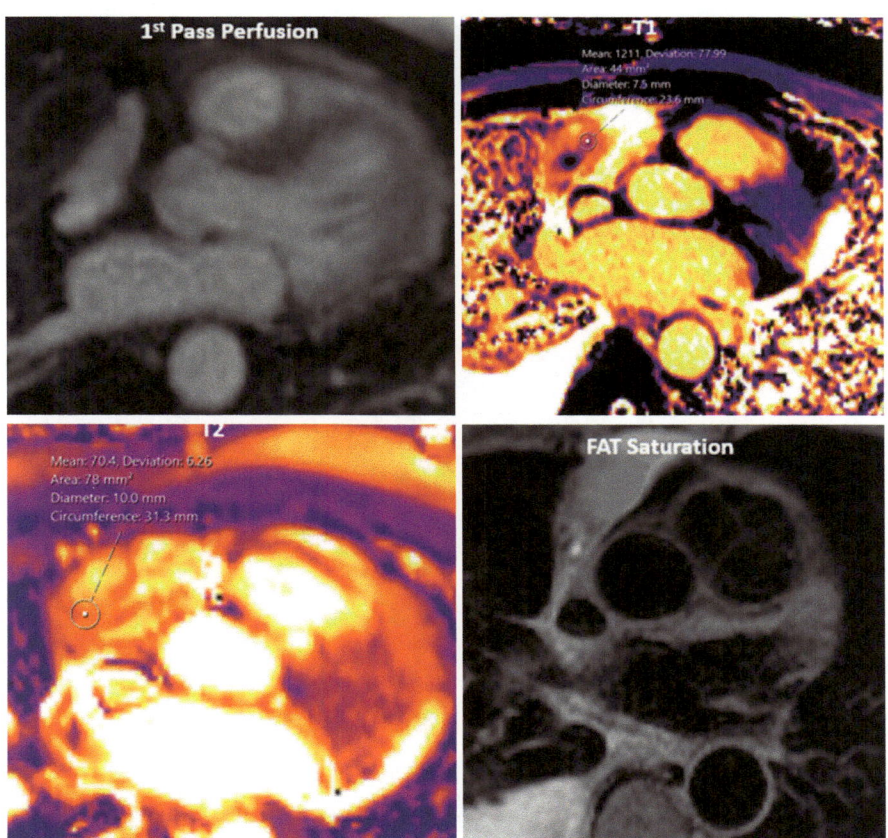

© The Author(s), under exclusive license to Springer Nature
Switzerland AG 2023
S. G. Al-Kindi, S. E. Janus, *Cardiac MRI Certification Exam*,
https://doi.org/10.1007/978-3-031-25966-1_5

(A) Pericardial cyst
(B) Pericardial fatty tumor
(C) Pericardial thrombus
(D) Normal pericardium

The correct answer is A. The images demonstrate a 4.4 × 2.2 cm cystic mass that appears to be in continuity with the pericardium and gives rise to extrinsic compression of the RA. The mass exhibits isointense T1 and mildly hyperintense T2 signals. There is no uptake on first pass perfusion (Figure A), therefore likely consistent with pericardial cyst [1]. A pericardial fatty tumor would be suppressed on fat saturation. A pericardial thrombus should have hypointense T1 and T2 signals and is less likely to be present in the pericardium.

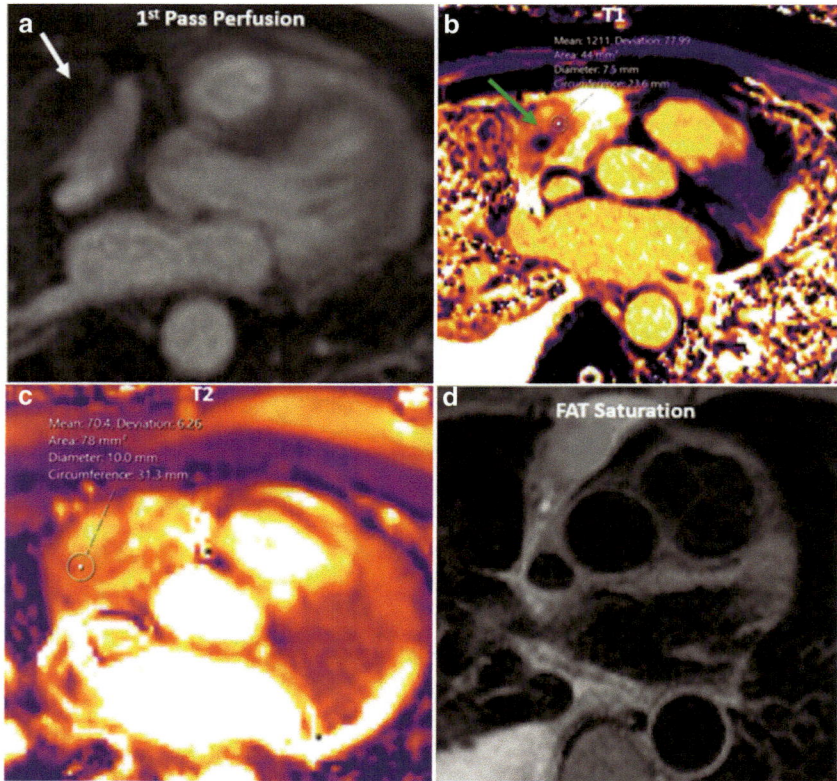

First pass perfusion with white arrow demonstrating a no contrast uptake. B- T1 demonstrating isointense mass. C- T2 demonstrating a mildly hyperintense signal, D- T1 turbospin echo with fat saturation showing no suppression of the signal from the mass

79. Where is the mass located?

TI Vibe

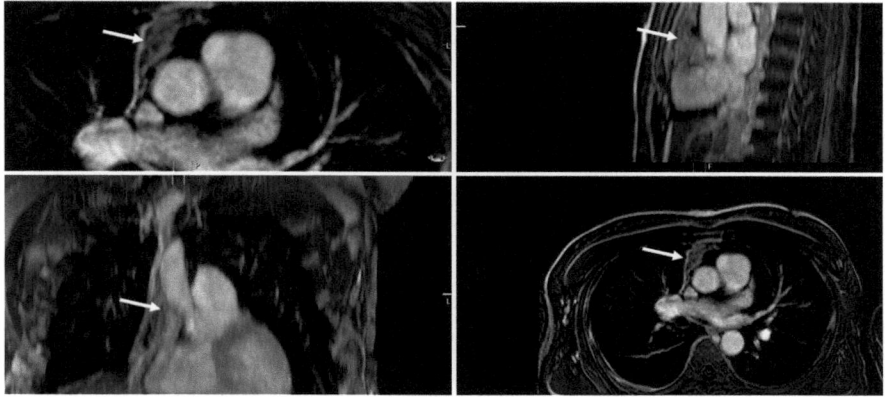

(A) Mediastinum
(B) Pericardium
(C) Pulmonary artery
(D) Superior vena cava

The correct answer is B. The mass is located within the pericardium. This particular mass is a pericardial cyst. However, the mass is surrounded by the pericardial layer so within the pericardium [2].

80. The following images most likely demonstrate?

PSIR Delayed Enhancement Imaging

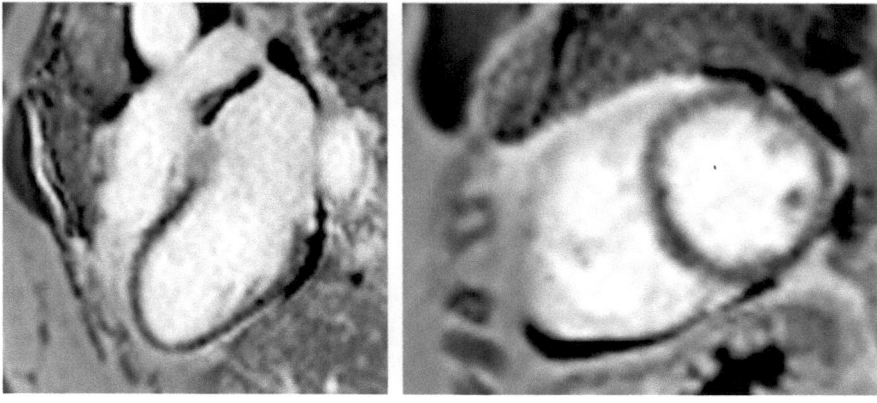

(A) Myocarditis
(B) Infarct
(C) Infiltration
(D) Pericarditis

The correct answer is D. On this delayed enhancement imaging, there is small pericardial effusion with pericardial enhancement, consistent with pericarditis [3]. There is no myocardial enhancement to suggest myocarditis, infarction, or infiltration.

PSIR Delayed Enhancement Imaging

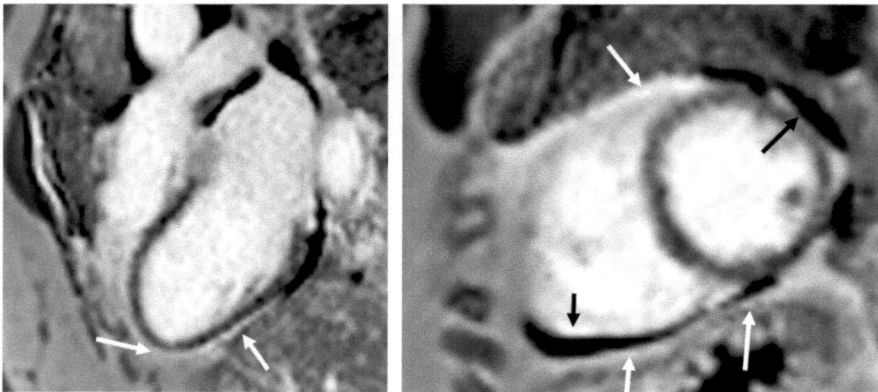

PSIR Delayed Enhancement Imaging- White arrows demonstrating pericardial inflammation/enhancement. Black arrows demonstrating pericardial fluid/effusion

81. What is displayed in the image below?

PSIR Delayed Imaging

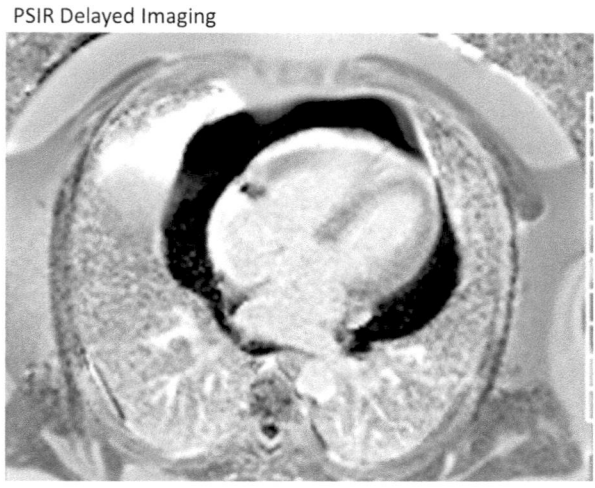

(A) Large pericardial fat pad
(B) Large pericardial effusion
(C) Pericardial tumor
(D) Pericardial mass

The correct answer is B. The PSIR delayed imaging shows a large pericardial effusion which appears black on PSIR images due to a long T1 signal and without uptake of gadolinium. These are often obvious on SSFP imaging, though differentiation between epicardial fat and pericardial effusion can be difficult and requires additional imaging. PSIR can differentiate between epicardial fat (bright) and pericardial effusion (black). A pericardial mass or tumor would be a discrete mass, not circumferential like the pericardial fluid above.

82. The following image is most consistent with?

Delayed Enhancement MAG High Res   Delayed Enhancement PSIR High Res

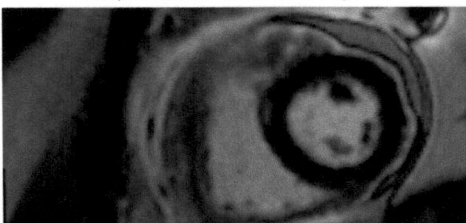 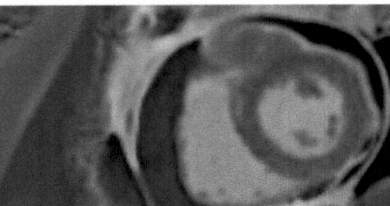

(A) Pericardial enhancement
(B) Myocardial infarction
(C) Myocarditis
(D) Pericardial fat

The correct answer is A. The delayed enhancement imaging demonstrates pericardial effusion with significant pericardial enhancement which is consistent with a diagnosis of acute pericarditis [4]. The pericardium is thickened [5]. There is no evidence of myocardial enhancement to suggest myocarditis. PSIR imaging separates water and fat to demonstrate effusion vs pericardial enhancement [6].

Delayed Enhancement MAG High Res   Delayed Enhancement PSIR High Res

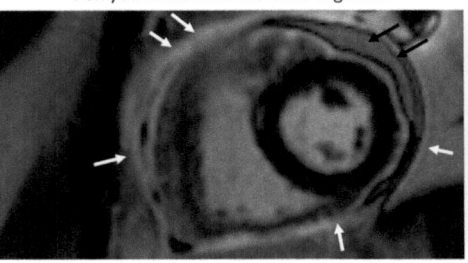 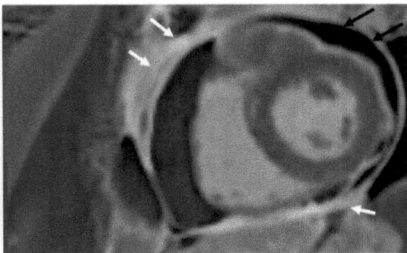

Delayed Enhancement Imaging demonstrating thick, inflammed pericardium (white arrows), with small pericardial effusion (black arrows).

83. The following images are most consistent with what diagnosis?

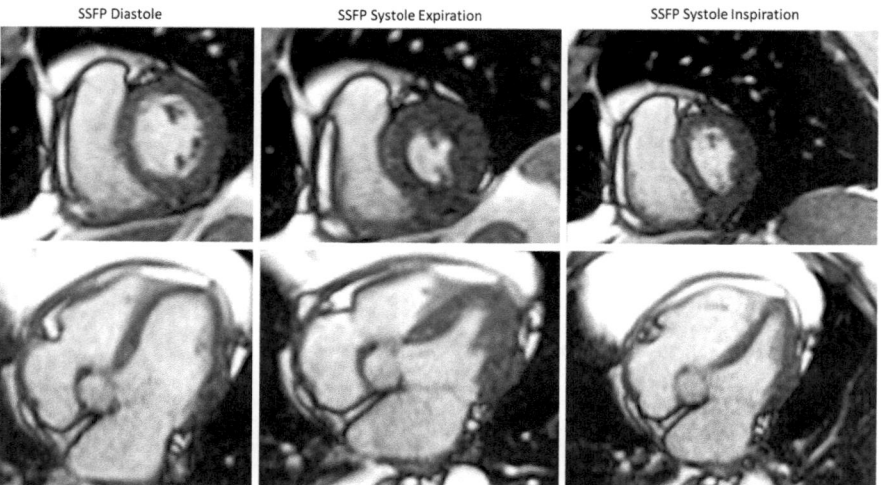

(A) Cor pulmonale
(B) Acute pulmonary embolism
(C) Superior vena cava syndrome
(D) Ventricular interdependence

The correct answer is D. The images demonstrate a diagnosis of constrictive pericarditis. There is ventricular interdependence [7]. The steady-state free precession images demonstrate a significant "septal shudder" or septal shift of the septum into the left ventricle on inspiration/free breathing. This occurs secondary to elevated intrapericardial pressures (tamponade) or can occur when there is thickened pericardium that restricts filling. There are no signs of a dilated pulmonary artery, which can be seen in cor pulmonale. There is no right ventricular enlargement or signs of McConnell's sign to suggest pulmonary embolism. The superior vena cava is not seen and does not demonstrate occlusion.

84. What is the likely diagnosis?

PSIR Delayed enhancement

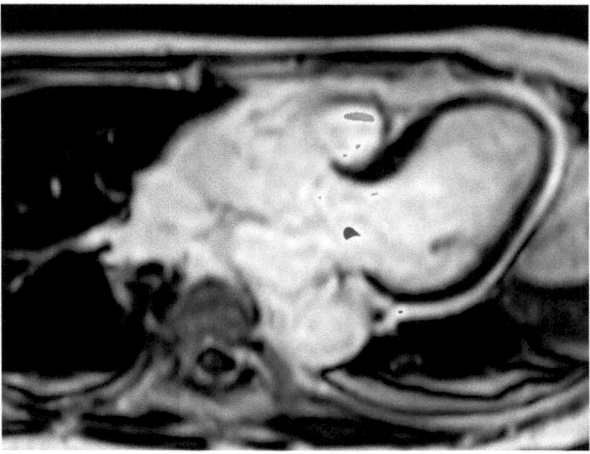

(A) Pericardial enhancement
(B) LAD infarction
(C) Aortic dissection
(D) Myocarditis

The correct answer is A. The pericardium shows diffuse enhancement increasing the likelihood this is acute pericarditis [8]. There is no enhancement within the myocardium to suggest infarct. There is no indication of dissection within the aorta. There is no enhancement in the mid-myocardium to suggest myocarditis.

PSIR Delayed enhancement

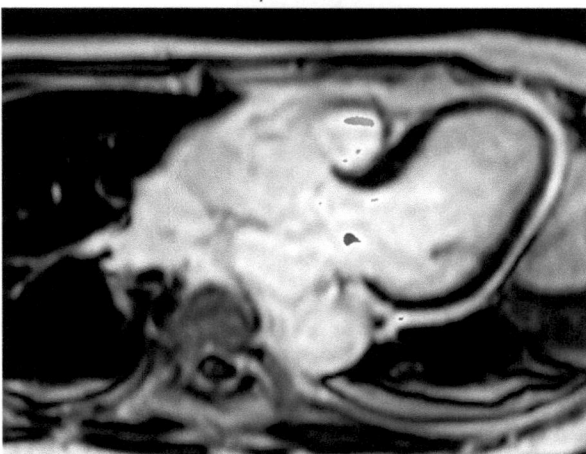

PSIR Delayed enhancement- showing diffuse enhancement in the pericardium, likely reflecting pericardial inflammation.

85. What is the most likely diagnosis?

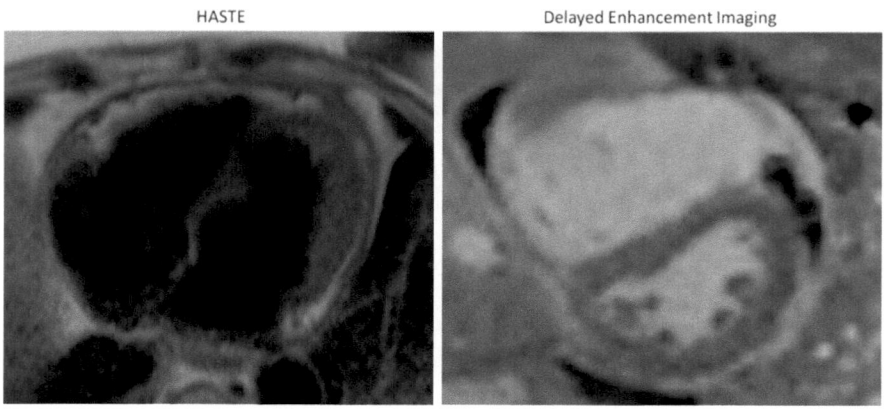

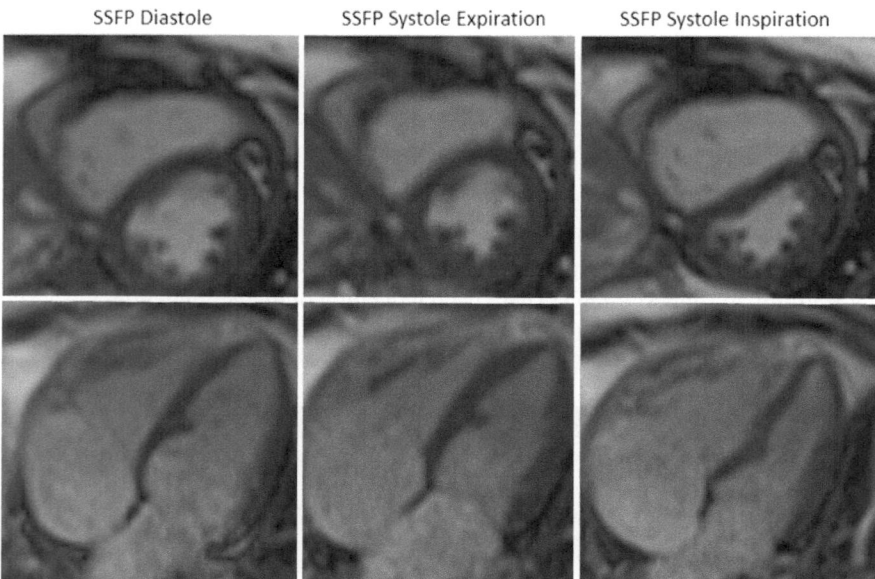

(A) Constrictive pericarditis
(B) Tamponade
(C) Myxoma
(D) ARVC

The correct answer is A, constrictive pericarditis. The images demonstrate a thickened pericardium. There is enhancement of the pericardium on delayed enhancement imaging. The SSFP images demonstrate inspiration septal shudder/interventricular interdependence with bowing of the right ventricle into the left ventricle during inspiration [9].

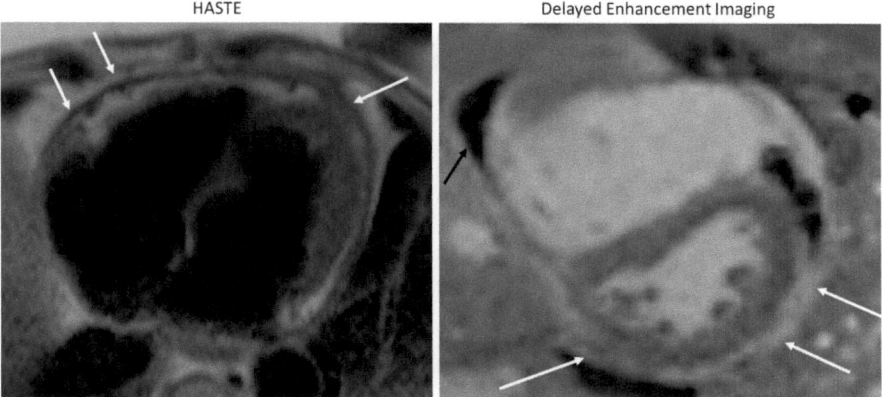

HASTE- Haste imaging demonstrating thickened pericardium (white arrows). The delayed enhancement imaging demonstrates enhancement/inflammation throughout the pericardium (white arrows) with small effusion (black arrow)

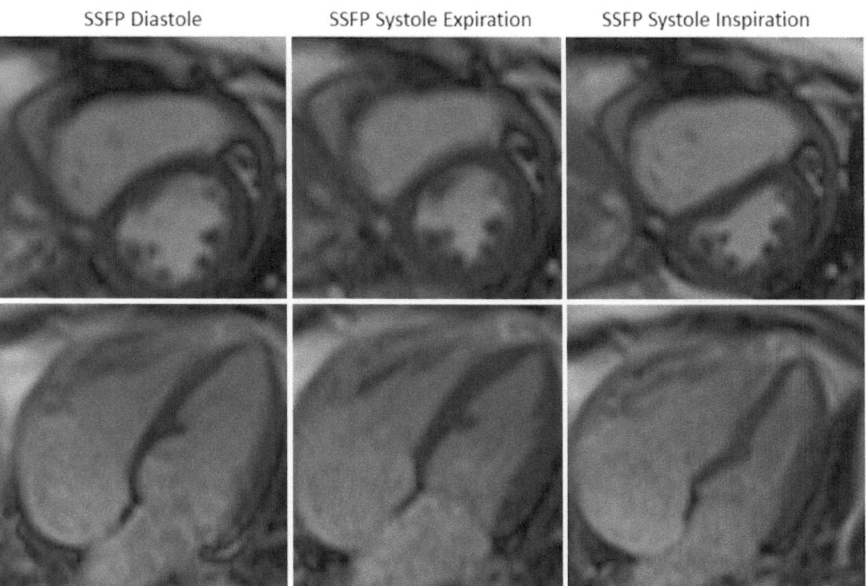

SSFP imaging demonstrating inspiration septal shift/shudder with bowing of the right ventricle during inspiration into the left ventricle, a sign of constrictive physiology.

86. What does the white arrow demonstrate?

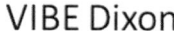

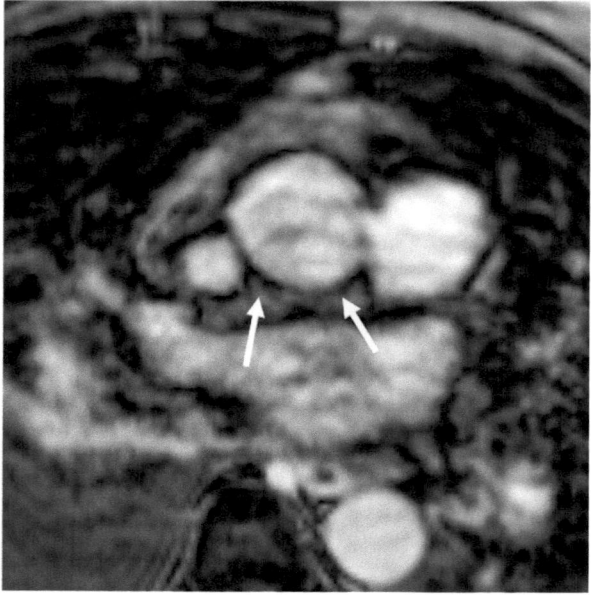

(A) Aortic dissection
(B) Enlarged esophagus
(C) Intramural hematoma
(D) Pericardial recess

The correct answer is D. The white arrows point to a pericardial recess of a normal structure in the heart [10]. The esophagus is normally located posterior to the left atrium/pulmonary veins. An intramural hematoma and aortic dissection would be seen within the aortic lumen which is not demonstrated here.

References

1. Hoey ETD, Shahid M, Watkin RW. Computed tomography and magnetic resonance imaging evaluation of pericardial disease. Quant Imaging Med Surg. 2016;6(3):274–84. https://doi.org/10.21037/qims.2016.01.03.
2. Meredith A. Pericardial cyst. Treasure Island. 2022.
3. Khandaker MH, Espinosa RE, Nishimura RA, Sinak LJ, Hayes SN, Melduni RM, Oh JK. Pericardial disease: diagnosis and management. Mayo Clin Proc. 2010;85(6):572–93. https://doi.org/10.4065/mcp.2010.0046.

4. Aldweib N, Farah V, Biederman RWW. Clinical utility of cardiac magnetic resonance imaging in pericardial diseases. Curr Cardiol Rev. 2018;14(3):200–12. https://doi.org/10.2174/1573403X14666180619104515.
5. Janus SE, Hoit BD. Effusive–constrictive pericarditis in the spectrum of pericardial compressive syndromes. Heart. 2021;107(6):450–5. https://doi.org/10.1136/heartjnl-2020-316664.
6. Kellman P, Hernando D, Shah S, Zuehlsdorff S, Jerecic R, Liang Z-P, Arai AE. 1025 Multi-echo dixon fat and water separation method for detecting fibro-fatty infiltration in the myocardium. J Cardiovasc Magn Reson. 2008;10(S1):A150, 1532-429X-10-S1-A150. https://doi.org/10.1186/1532-429X-10-S1-A150
7. Moseley A, Mazur W, Ahmad S. Cardiac magnetic resonance imaging in unclear cases of ventricular interdependence: a case series. Eur Heart J - Case Rep. 2021;5(7):ytab223. https://doi.org/10.1093/ehjcr/ytab223
8. Mikolich JR. New diagnostic criteria for acute pericarditis: a cardiac MRI perspective; 7.
9. Klein AL, Abbara S, Agler DA, Appleton CP, Asher CR, Hoit B, Hung J, Garcia MJ, Kronzon I, Oh JK, Rodriguez ER, Schaff HV, Schoenhagen P, Tan CD, White RD. American Society of Echocardiography Clinical Recommendations for Multimodality Cardiovascular Imaging of Patients with Pericardial Disease. J Am Soc Echocardiogr. 2013;26(9):965–1012.e15. https://doi.org/10.1016/j.echo.2013.06.023.
10. Truong MT, Erasmus JJ, Gladish GW, Sabloff BS, Marom EM, Madewell JE, Chasen MH, Munden RF. Anatomy of pericardial recesses on multidetector CT: implications for oncologic imaging. Am J Roentgenol. 2003;181(4):1109–13. https://doi.org/10.2214/ajr.181.4.1811109.

Chapter 6
Valvular Disease

87. Calculating the amount of mitral regurgitation requires:

(A) Aortic forward flow—left ventricle stroke volume
(B) Left ventricular stroke volume—aortic forward flow
(C) Right ventricular stroke volume—aortic forward flow
(D) Left ventricular stroke volume—pulmonary forward flow

The correct answer is B. Quantification of the standard method of indirect quantification of mitral regurgitation involves subtracting the aortic forward flow from the left ventricular stroke volume (LVSV—AoFF). Recent methods also include left ventricle systolic volume minus right ventricle systolic volume [1]. A is incorrect because this is reversed (aortic flow should be subtracted from the left ventricular stroke volume). C is incorrect because the right ventricle should not be compared to the aortic forward flow. Lastly, D is incorrect as the pulmonary flow is upstream from the left ventricle and not always equivalent to the aortic flow.

© The Author(s), under exclusive license to Springer Nature
Switzerland AG 2023
S. G. Al-Kindi, S. E. Janus, *Cardiac MRI Certification Exam*,
https://doi.org/10.1007/978-3-031-25966-1_6

88. Match the cusps with the correct name.

Steady State Free Precession

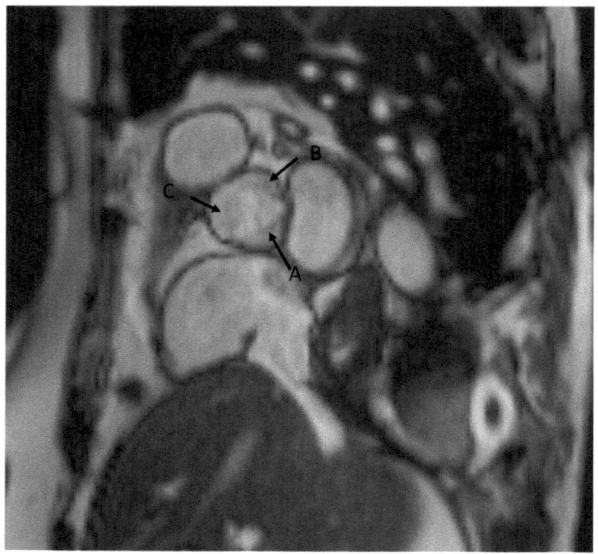

(A) A—Non-coronary cusp, B—Right coronary cusp, C—Left coronary cusp
(B) A—Non-coronary cusp, B—Left coronary cusp, C—Right coronary cusp
(C) A—Left coronary cusp, B—Non-coronary cusp, C—Right coronary cusp
(D) A—Right coronary cusp, B—Non-coronary cusp, C—Left coronary cusp
(E) A—Left coronary cusp, B—Right coronary cusp, C—Non-coronary cusp

The correct answer is B. The non-coronary cusp always points toward the inter-atrial septum. The right coronary cusp is usually the anterior structure, while the left coronary is usually posterior. Therefore, choice B is the correct answer [2].

Steady State Free Precession

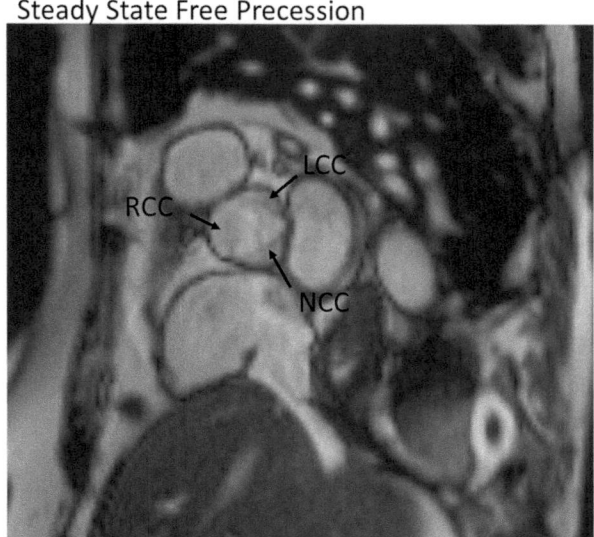

89. What can be done to obtain better visualization of the valve?

Steady State Free Precession

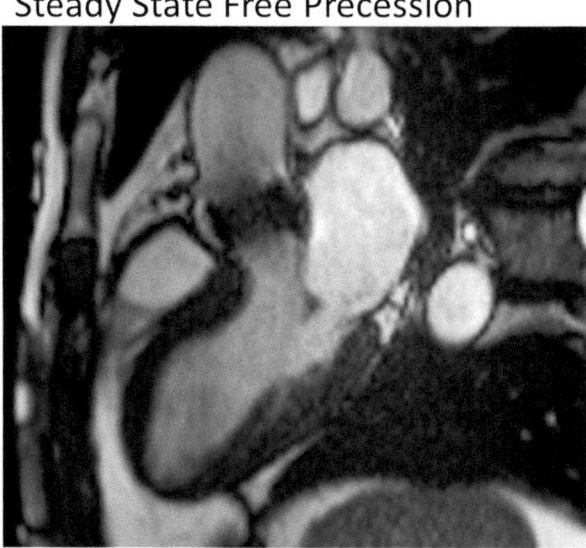

(A) Change to Gradient Echo (GRE) sequence
(B) Change to turbo spin echo
(C) Decrease flip angle
(D) Increase flip angle

The correct answer is A. When steady-state free precession images are having interaction with valves or grafts, gradient echo images provide better visualization [3]. Changing the flip angle will not change the quality of visualization of the valve.

90. How would one calculate the amount of tricuspid regurgitation?

SSFP 4 Chamber

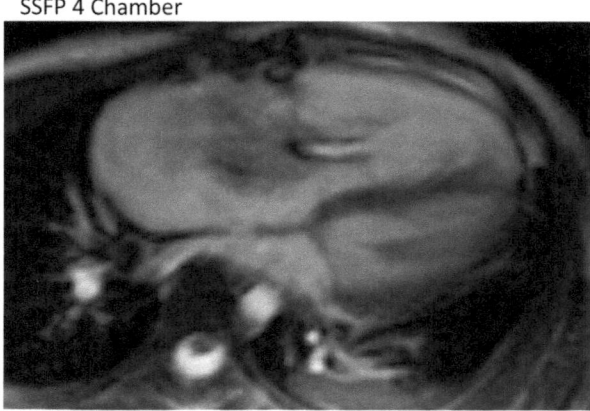

(A) Right ventricular stroke volume—pulmonary flow volume
(B) Pulmonary flow volume—right ventricular stroke volume
(C) Right ventricular stroke volume—left ventricular stroke volume
(D) pulmonic flow volume—left ventricular stroke volume

The correct answer is A. In order to calculate tricuspid regurgitation, we typically use the right ventricular stroke volume subtracting the pulmonary flow volume to calculate the regurgitant volume (indirect method) [4].

91. What is the likely diagnosis?

SSFP Short axis of Aortic Valve

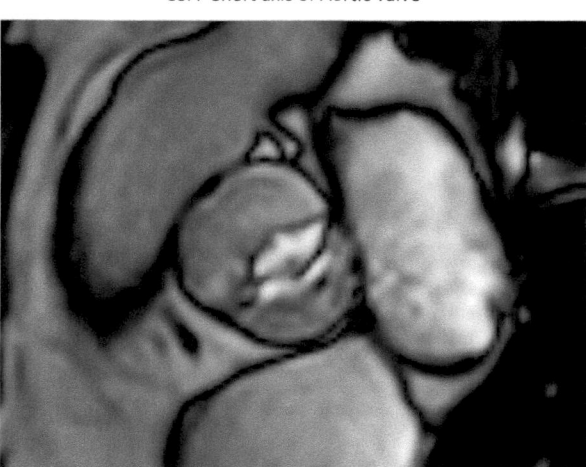

(A) Fusion of the non-coronary and right coronary cusp
(B) Fusion of the non-coronary and left coronary cusp
(C) Fusion of the left and right coronary cusp
(D) Quadricuspid aortic valve
(E) Mono-cuspid aortic valve

The correct answer is C. There is a fusion of the left and the right coronary cusp [5].

SSFP Short axis of Aortic Valve

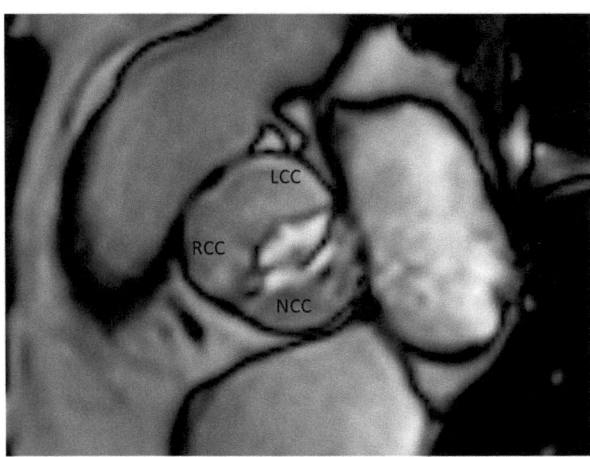

92. How does one calculate the regurgitant fraction of aortic insufficiency?

(A) (Aortic flow—LV stroke volume)/Aortic flow volume
(B) (LV stroke volume—Aortic flow volume)/LV stroke volume
(C) Aortic reverse flow diastolic volume/Aortic forward systolic volume
(D) Aortic reverse flow diastolic volume/LV stroke volume systole

The correct answer is C. Aortic reverse flow diastolic volume/Aortic forward systolic volume gives the amount of aortic regurgitation [6]. (LV stroke volume—Aortic flow volume)/LV stroke volume is the amount of mitral regurgitation. The other two are not correct formulas [7].

93. Calculate the amount of pulmonic insufficiency.

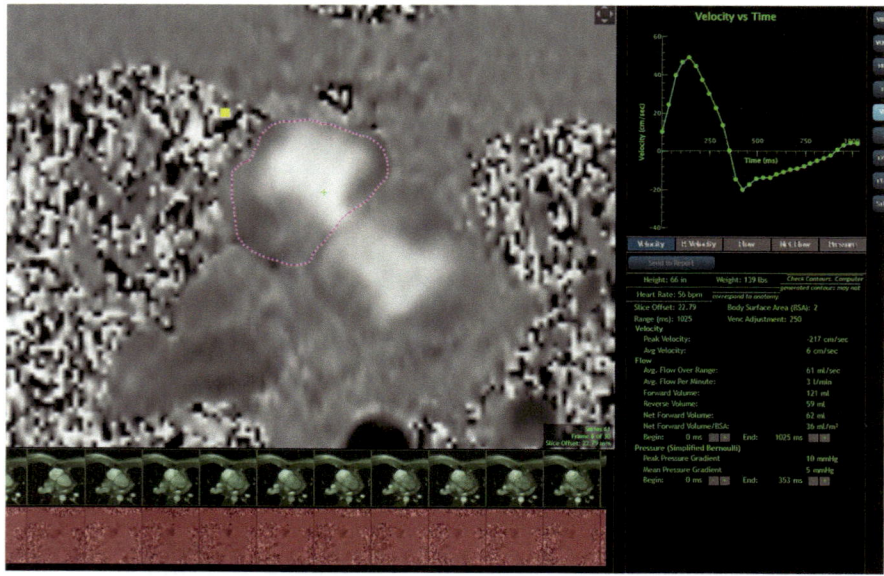

Avg Flow Over Range 61 ml/s, Avg Flow per minute 3 L/min, Forward volume 121 ml, reverse volume 59 ml, Net forward 62 ml/min, net forward per BSA 36 ml/m^2, Peak gradient 10 mmHg, Mean gradient 5 mmHg.

(A) Mild
(B) Moderate
(C) Severe
(D) Unable to calculate

The correct answer is B. The regurgitant volume is less than 60 ml, and the regurgitant fraction is 48% which falls into the moderate category. While approaching severe, by criteria this is still moderate for tricuspid regurgitation.

Tricuspid regurgitation			
Degree	Mild	Moderate	Severe
Regurgitant volume (ml)	<30	30–59	≥60
Regurgitant fraction (RF%)	<30	30–50	>50

Regurgitant volumes are measured directly and calculated by Regurgitant fraction (%) = volume of TR (ml)/RVSV (ml)

94. Which of the following is moderate tricuspid insufficiency?

(A) Regurgitant volume 28 ml, regurgitant fraction 28%
(B) Regurgitant volume 35 ml, regurgitant fraction 28%

(C) Regurgitant volume 58 ml, regurgitant fraction 48%
(D) Regurgitant volume 68 ml, regurgitant fraction 51%

The most correct answer is C. Tricuspid regurgitation is graded based on the scale below [8].

Tricuspid regurgitation			
Degree	Mild	Moderate	Severe
Regurgitant volume (ml)	<30	30–59	≥60
Regurgitant fraction (RF%)	<30	30–50	>50
Regurgitant volumes are measured directly and calculated by Regurgitant fraction (%) = volume of TR (ml)/RVSV (ml)			

95. Which of the following describes moderate aortic insufficiency?

(A) Regurgitant volume 28 ml, regurgitant fraction 28%
(B) Regurgitant volume 35 ml, regurgitant fraction 28%
(C) Regurgitant volume 48 ml, regurgitant fraction 48%
(D) Regurgitant volume 68 ml, regurgitant fraction 51%

The best answer is C. Aortic insufficiency is based on the following chart. While B is close to the regurgitant volume of 35 ml, the regurgitant fraction is less than 30%, therefore C is a better answer [6].

Aortic regurgitation			
Degree	Mild	Moderate	Severe
Regurgitant volume (ml)	30	30–60	>60
Regurgitant fraction (RF%)	<30	30–50	>50
Regurgitant volumes are measured directly. Regurgitant fraction (%) = volume of AR (ml)/ LVSV (ml)			

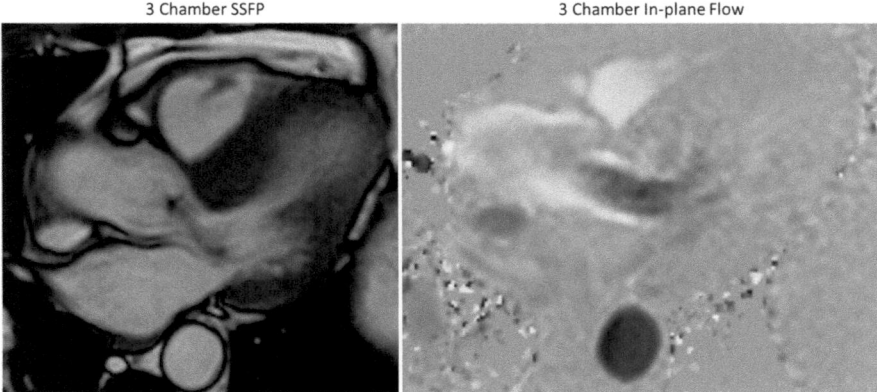

3 Chamber SSFP and in-plane flow demonstrating significant aortic insufficiency (white arrows)

96. Calculate the amount of aortic insufficiency.

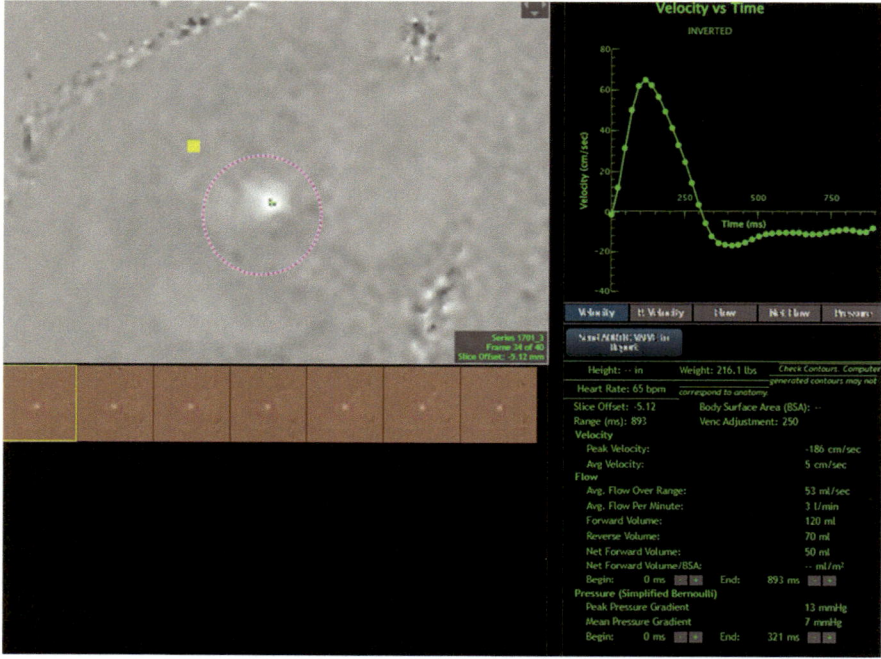

Forward volume 120 ml, reverse volume 70 ml, net forward flow 50 ml, Avg flow per minute 3 Lm/min.

(A) Regurgitant fraction 41%
(B) Regurgitant fraction 58%
(C) Regurgitant fraction 71%
(D) Regurgitant fraction 171%

The correct answer is B. The reverse volume divided by the forward volume gives the regurgitant fraction, in this case 70 ml/120 ml which equals 58% [6].

97. What is the most likely diagnosis based on the below?

SSFP- Diastole   SSFP 4 Chamber- Diastole

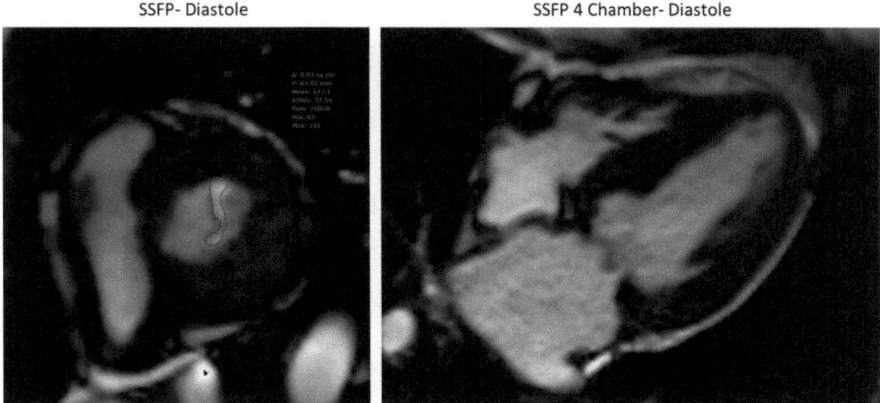

(A) Mitral stenosis
(B) Mitral insufficiency
(C) Atrial septal defect
(D) Epstein's anomaly

The correct answer is A. The SSFP images in diastole show severely restricted opening of the mitral valve in diastole with a valve area of 0.92 cm² [9].

SSFP- Diastole   SSFP 4 Chamber- Diastole

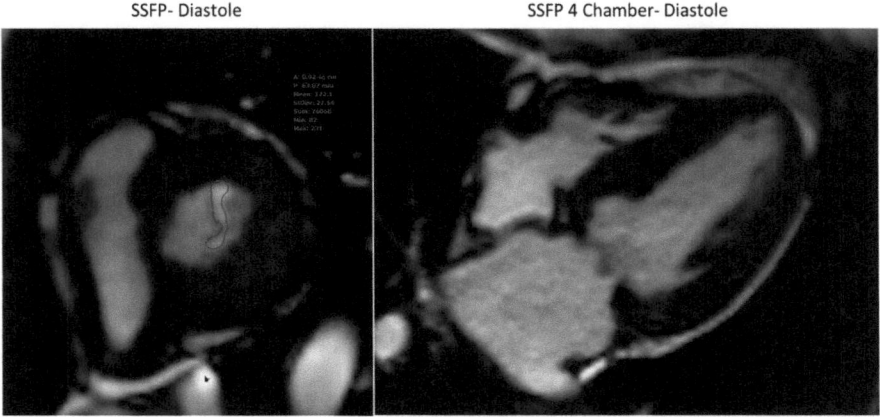

SSFP- Diastole images showing severely restricted opening of the mitral valve with valve area <1.0cm2 by planimetry.

Mitral Stenosis				
Degree	Normal	Mild	Moderate	Severe
MV area (cm2)	>2.0	1.5-2.0	1.0-1.5	<1.0

98. The best way to describe the following image is:

SSFP- 3 Chamber   SSFP

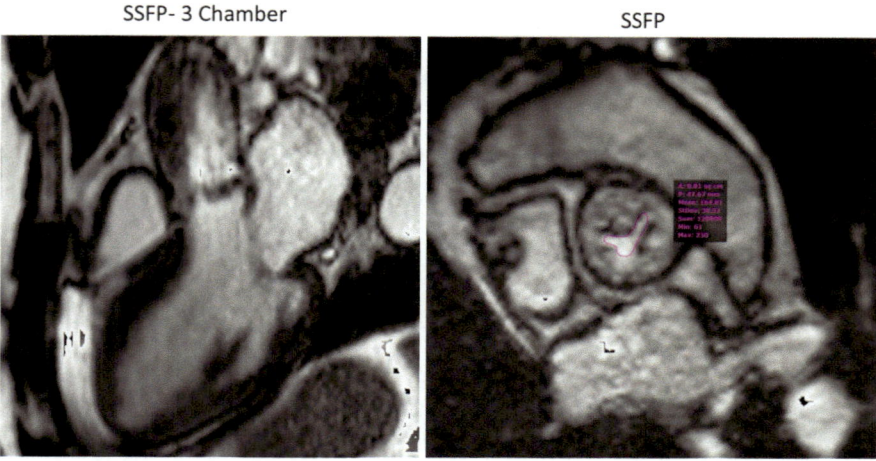

(A) Moderate aortic stenosis
(B) Severe aortic stenosis
(C) Sub-aortic membrane
(D) Supra-aortic valvular coarctation

The correct answer is B. The valve area by planimetry is 0.81 cm^2 which indicates severe aortic stenosis [10].

Aortic stenosis

Degree	Normal	Mild	Moderate	Severe
Valve area (cm²)	>2.0	1.6–2.0	1.0–1.5	<1.0
Peak pressure (mmHg)	–	<36	36–64	>64
Mean pressure (mmHg)	–	<25	25–40	>40
Peak velocity (m/s)	1	<3	3	>4

99. How would you describe aortic stenosis?

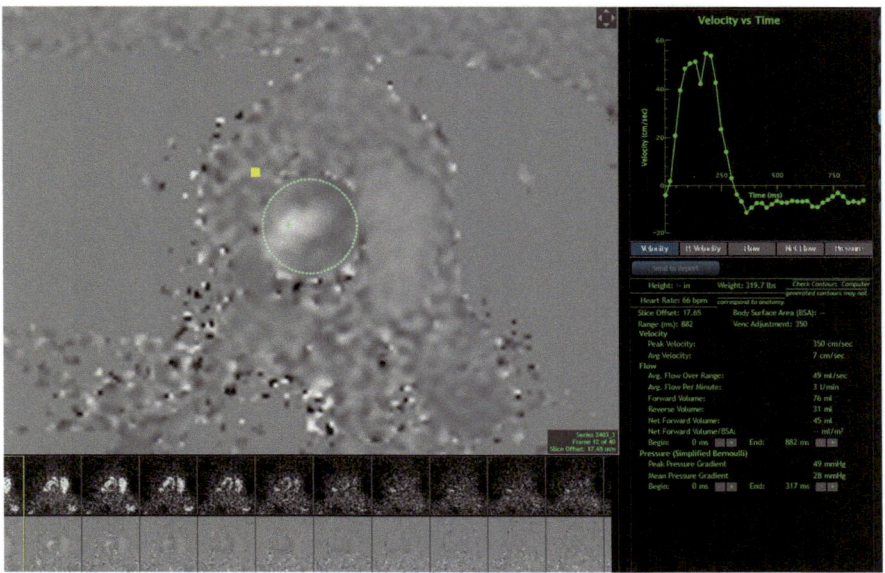

(A) Mild
(B) Moderate
(C) Severe
(D) Unable to tell

The correct answer is D. The graph of the peak velocity demonstrates aliasing and peak velocity not reached, so the gradients will be inaccurate. Aortic stenosis is defined as severe when the mean gradient is >40 mmHg [10].

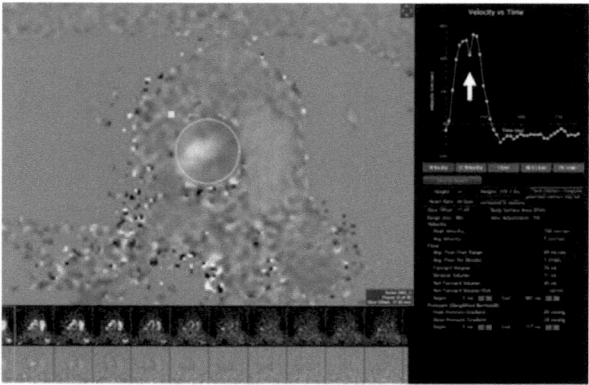

Velocity encoding demonstrating aliasing (white arrow) and therefore peak velocity not able to be obtained.

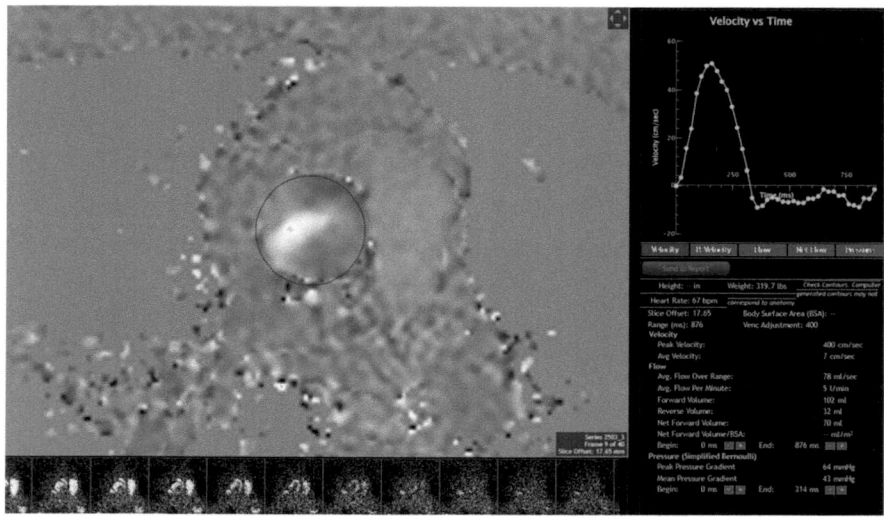

When the correct velocity encoding applied can see this is severe aortic stenosis with mean gradient >41mmHg.

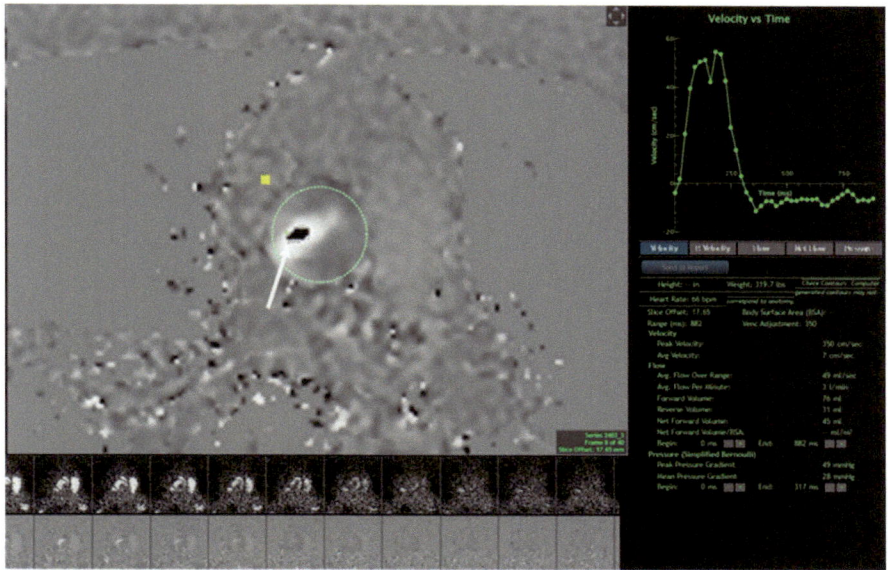

Velocity encoding demonstrating aliasing (white arrow) and therefore peak velocity not able to be obtained.

100. What is the diagnosis based on the following images?

SSFP 4 Chamber Systole

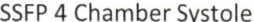

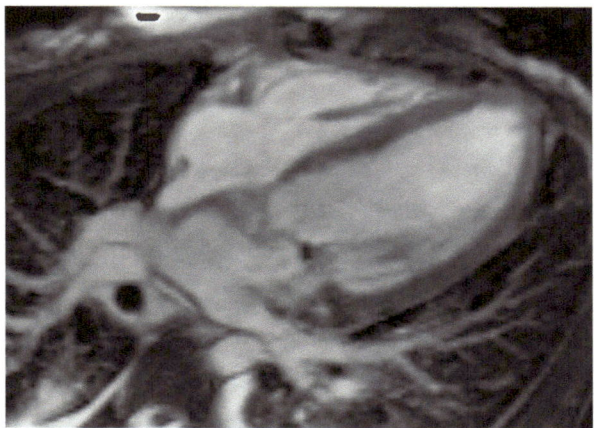

(A) Mitral valve endocarditis with regurgitation
(B) Tricuspid valve endocarditis with regurgitation
(C) Mitral valve stenosis
(D) Tricuspid valve stenosis

The correct answer is A. There is a small mass attached to the mitral valve. This mass is slightly mobile on CINE images and there is associated regurgitation [11].

SSFP 4 Chamber Systole

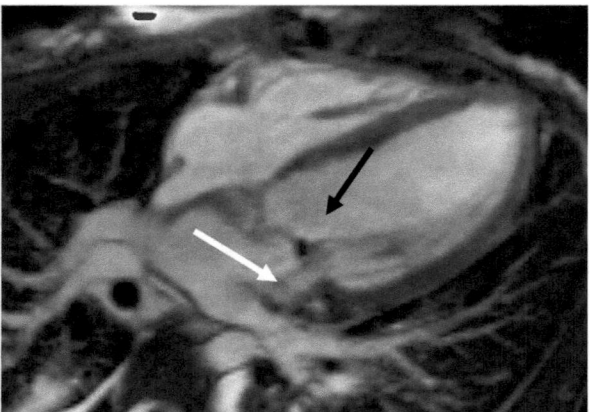

SSFP 4 Chamber Systole- Black arrow demonstrating the mitral valve mass and the white arrow demonstrating the regurgitation

References

1. Polte CL, Bech-Hanssen O, Johnsson ÅA, Gao SA, Lagerstrand KM. Mitral regurgitation quantification by cardiovascular magnetic resonance: a comparison of indirect quantification methods. Int J Cardiovasc Imaging. 2015;31(6):1223–31. https://doi.org/10.1007/s10554-015-0681-3.
2. Biederman R. Valvular heart disease. In: Radiol. Key. https://radiologykey.com/valvular-heart-disease-3/. Accessed 10 Jun 2022.
3. Cardiac MRI CM. Fast Gradient Echo. In: Fast Gradient Echo. 2022. https://cardiacmri.com/tech-guide/imaging-sequences/fast-gradient-echo/. Accessed 28 Aug 2022.
4. Lambert S. Regurgitant fraction. 2008.
5. Barker AJ, Markl M, Bürk J, Lorenz R, Bock J, Bauer S, Schulz-Menger J, von Knobelsdorff-Brenkenhoff F. Bicuspid aortic valve is associated with altered wall shear stress in the ascending aorta. Circ Cardiovasc Imaging. 2012;5(4):457–66. https://doi.org/10.1161/CIRCIMAGING.112.973370.
6. Cardiac MRI. Aortic Regurgitation. In: Card. MRI. 2022. https://cardiacmri.com/analysis-guide/aortic-valve-2/aorta/. Accessed 10 Jun 2022.
7. Myerson SG, d'Arcy J, Mohiaddin R, Greenwood JP, Karamitsos TD, Francis JM, Banning AP, Christiansen JP, Neubauer S. Aortic regurgitation quantification using cardiovascular magnetic resonance: association with clinical outcome. Circulation. 2012;126(12):1452–60. https://doi.org/10.1161/CIRCULATIONAHA.111.083600.
8. Cardiac MRI. Tricuspid Regurgitation. In: Card. MRI. 2022. https://cardiacmri.com/analysis-guide/tricuspid-valve/tricuspid-regurgitation/. Accessed 10 Jun 2022.

9. Cardiac MRI. Mitral stenosis. In: Card. MRI. 2022. https://cardiacmri.com/analysis-guide/mitral-valve/mitral-stenosis/. Accessed 10 Jun 2022.
10. Aortic Stenosis. In: Card. MRI. 2022. https://cardiacmri.com/analysis-guide/aortic-valve-2/aortic-stenosis-2/
11. Dursun M, Yilmaz S, Yilmaz E, Yilmaz R, Onur I, Oflaz H, Dindar A. The utility of cardiac MRI in diagnosis of infective endocarditis: preliminary results. Diagn Interv Radiol. 2015;21(1):28–33. https://doi.org/10.5152/dir.2014.14239.

Chapter 7
Masses

101. What is the likely cause of the following image?

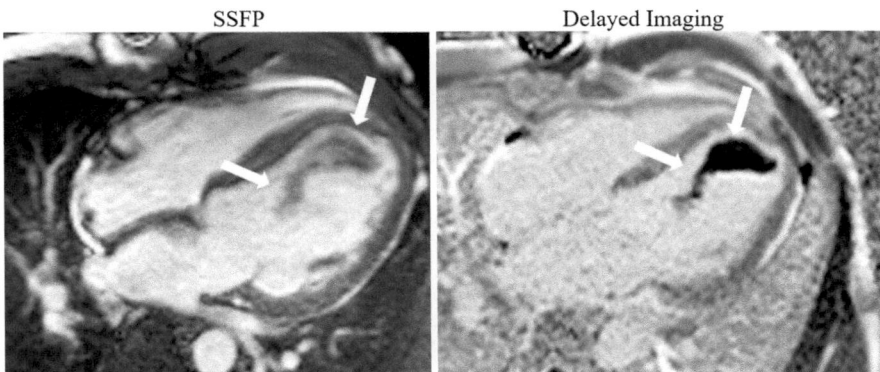

SSFP   Delayed Imaging

(A) LV thrombus
(B) Transmural infarction
(C) Blood dyscrasia
(D) Ingestion

The correct answer is A. The white arrows demonstrate a large left ventricular thrombus. B is incorrect due to no delayed enhancement in the myocardium [1]. There is no evidence of blood dyscrasia in this patient. See supplemental video 1.

S. G. Al-Kindi, S. E. Janus, *Cardiac MRI Certification Exam*,
https://doi.org/10.1007/978-3-031-25966-1_7

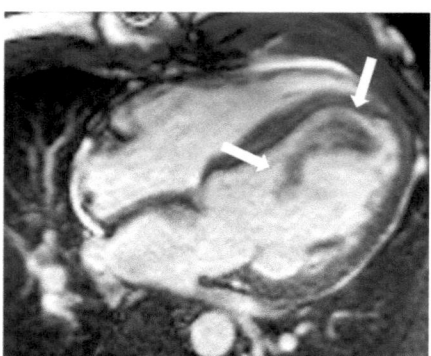
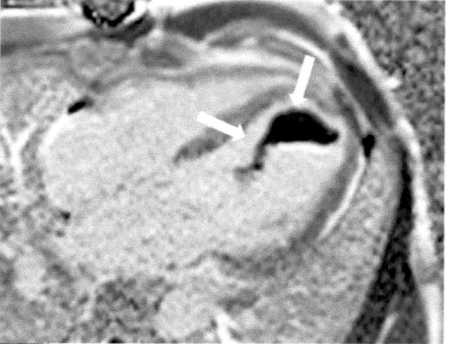

Figure 5A- White arrows demonstrate large left ventricular thrombus on cine (SSFP) imaging

Figure 5B- White arrows demonstrate large left ventricular thrombus on delayed enhancement imaging

102. The best series to evaluate left ventricular thrombus involves:

(A) Gradient spin echo
(B) Steady-state free precession
(C) Post-gadolinium imaging with long TI time
(D) Turbo Spin Echo

The correct answer is D. As seen below, delayed enhancement imaging with long TI time readily demonstrates LV thrombus easily to the viewer [2]. Cine-CMR (SSFP and GRE) increased the diagnostic efficiency for echocardiographic thrombus identification in this group, with sensitivity increasing from 50% by echocardiography to 75% by cine-CM [3]. However, late gadolinium imaging demonstrated the highest sensitivity and specificity of 88% and 99%, respectively [4].

103. What is the abnormality present in the following image?

Axial HASTE

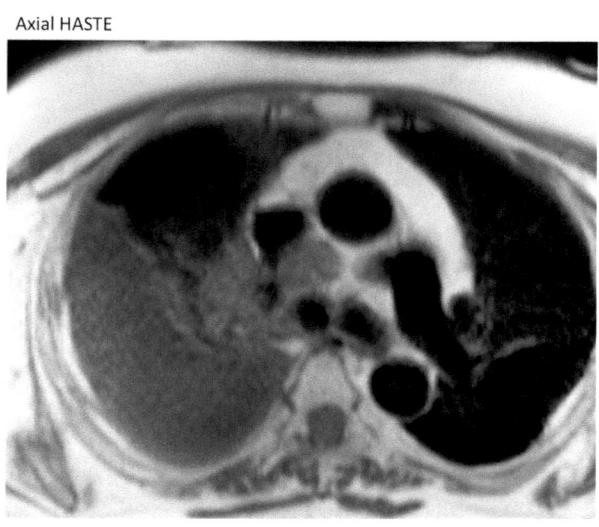

(A) Hepatomegaly
(B) Splenomegaly
(C) Lung mass and effusion
(D) Pulmonary artery embolism

The correct answer is C. The axial haste demonstrates a large left pleural effusion and mediastinal mass. Non-cardiac findings are very important to recognize and commonly present on HASTE anatomical or scout images [5]. This is not hepatomegaly, as we can see the aorta and pulmonary artery meaning the image is quite high in the chest. The spleen should be located on the left side of the body. The pulmonary artery would be better visualized if the intent was to demonstrate a pulmonary artery embolism.

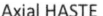

Axial HASTE

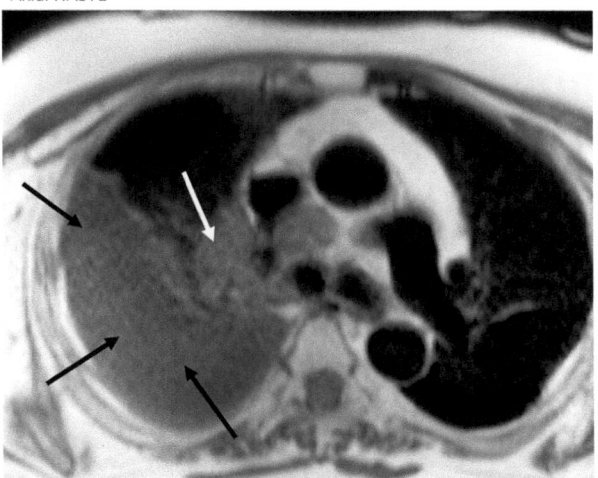

Axial HASTE demonstrating large right pleural effusion (black arrows) and mass located in the mediastinum (white arrows).

104. The following image is most consistent with:

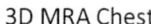

3D MRA Chest

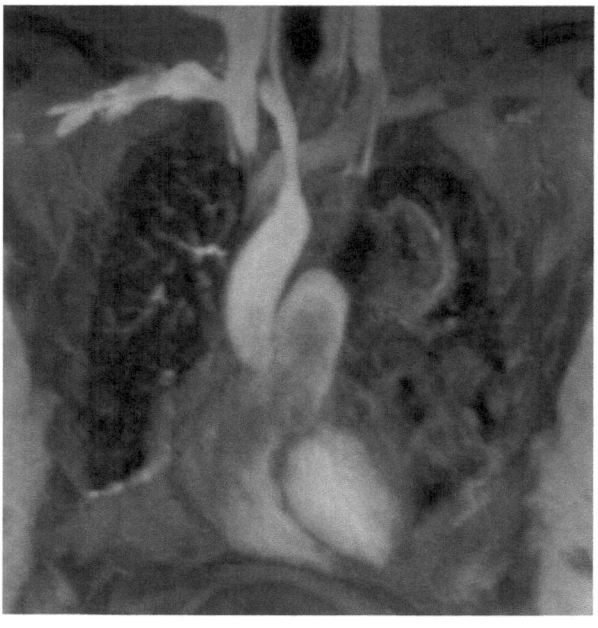

(A) Liver mass
(B) Mediastinal mass
(C) Diaphragmatic mass
(D) Kidney mass

The correct answer is B. The mediastinum demonstrates a large mass that has both hyper-enhancement along with a necrotic core. The mass is beginning to enhance on this early MRA image [6]. There are no liver or diaphragmatic lesions seen. A kidney mass would more likely be seen in the abdomen and most likely on scout images.

3D MRA Chest

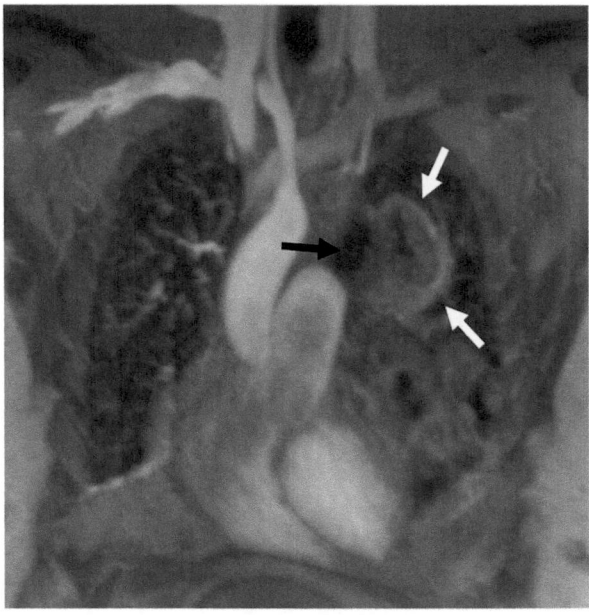

White arrows demonstrating hyper
enhancement and gadolinium uptake in the
rim. The black arrows represent the
necrotic core

105. What is the most likely diagnosis?

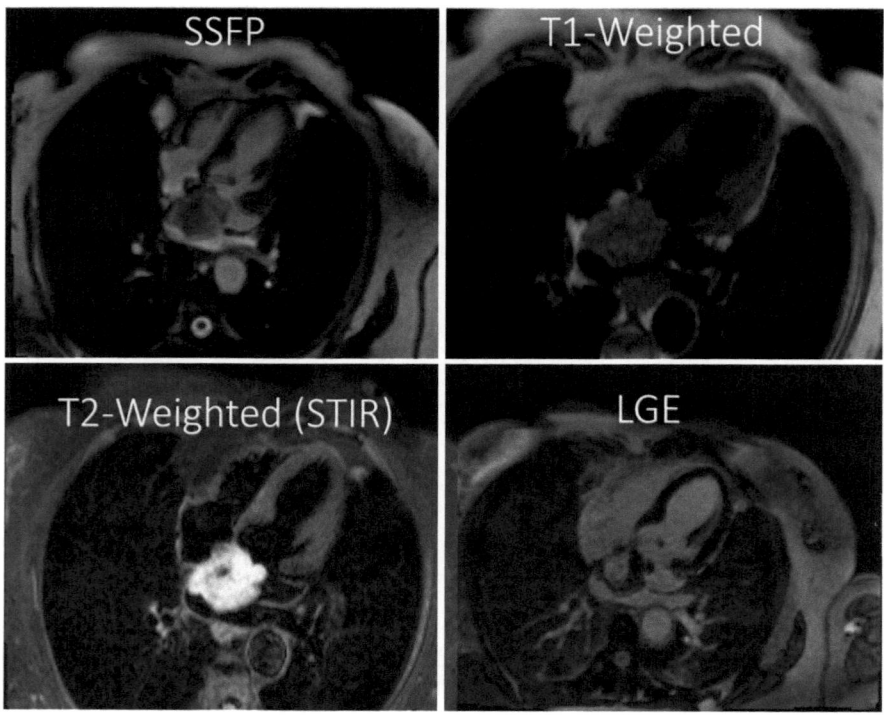

(A) Atrial myxoma
(B) Pericardial tumor
(C) Artifact
(D) Lipoma

   The correct answer is A. The mass demonstrates isointense on T1, high T2, and heterogenous LGE. This is consistent with atrial myxoma [7]. There is no mass demonstrated in the pericardium. The tumor would be low on T1 if consistent with lipoma.

106. What is the most likely diagnosis based on the following images?

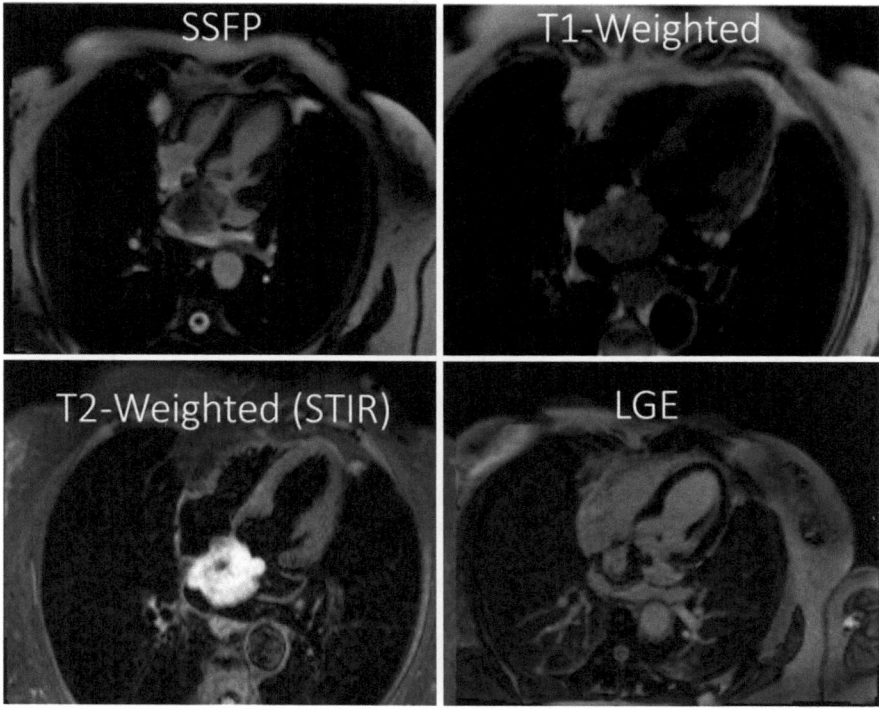

(A) Myxoma
(B) Metastatic melanoma
(C) Thrombus in transit
(D) Ventricular septal defect with closure device

The correct answer is B. The 4 chamber demonstrates a mass in the right ventricle, which showed increased T2 signals and heterogenous uptake TI600 with a necrotic core. This makes the most likely diagnosis of metastatic melanoma [8]. A thrombus would not take up gadolinium. A ventricular septal defect closure device would demonstrate artifact and be on both sides of the interventricular septum. A myxoma would more likely occur in the atrium.

107. The most likely diagnosis is:

T1 value of mass—227 ms, Myocardium T1-1261 ms
T2 Value Mass—116 ms, Myocardium 55.8 ms

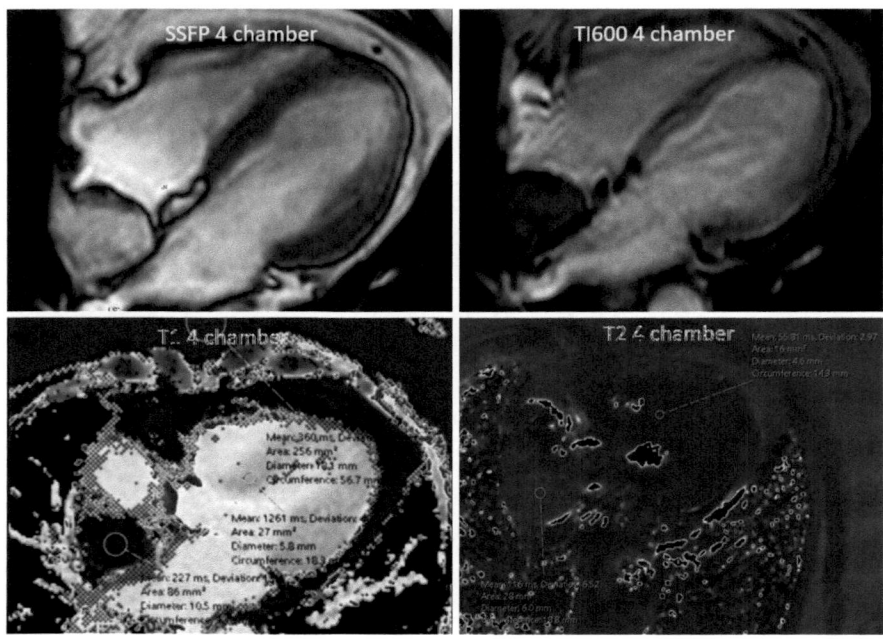

(A) Myxoma
(B) Thrombus
(C) Lipoma
(D) Pericardial cyst

The correct answer is C. The mass demonstrates elevated T2 value and isointense T1 value. There is no uptake of gadolinium making this likely lipoma or fatty tumor [9]. A myxoma would be a mixed uptake of gadolinium. A thrombus would be low on T1 and T2 values. A pericardial cyst would be high T2 and high T1 values and would be outside the pericardium, not within the right atrium.

Cardiac mass	T1-weighted imaging	T2-weighted imaging	Contrast enhancement (Late gadolinium enhancement)
Thrombus	Low (higher if more recent)	Low (higher if more recent)	No uptake
Pericardial cyst	Low	High (reflecting fluid)	No uptake
Myxoma	Isointense	High	Heterogeneous/Mixed
Lipoma	Isointense	High	No uptake
Lymphoma	Isointense	Isointense	No/very mild uptake
Metastatic Disease	Low	High	Heterogeneous/Mixed
Sarcoma (Rhabdomyo)	Isointense	Isointense	Heterogeneous/Mixed
Sarcoma (Angio)	Heterogeneous	Heterogeneous	Heterogeneous

Source: MRI Imaging of Cardiac Tumors and Masses: A review of methods and clinical applications <https://doi.org/10.1148/radiol.13121239>

108. The following images demonstrate:

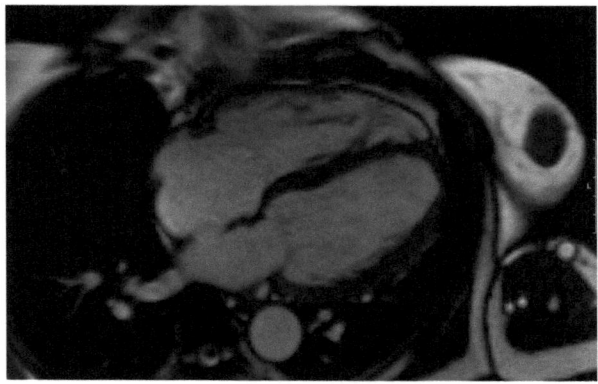

(A) Dilated pulmonary artery
(B) Aortic dissection
(C) Pneumonia
(D) Breast mass

The image demonstrates a mass in the left breast. This was actually caused by an artifact from a body piercing, however, it is important to examine images for breast masses [10]. There are no signs of an aortic dissection in the ascending or descending aorta. There is no dilation of the pulmonary artery. There is no pneumonia or consolidation in the lung fields.

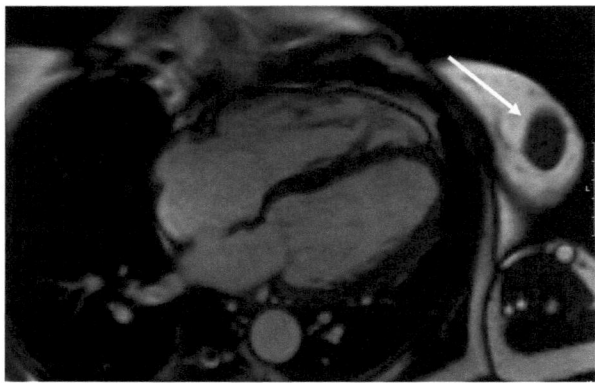

109. How often do extracardiac incidental findings are seen on cardiac MRI?

(A) Incidental findings are rare <0.5% of the time
(B) Cardiac images have a very limited field of view, therefore, incidental findings are not likely
(C) Significant incidental findings can occur in as many as 1 out of 10 cases
(D) Significant incidental findings occur in over 30% of cases

Significant extracardiac incidental findings can occur in as many as 1 in 10 cases. Research shows around 13–16% have major incidental findings [11]. Lung and liver are the most common sites for incidental findings. Scout images and sagittal/coronal views often contain other organs, which can demonstrate non-cardiac pathology.

110. What is seen in the images below?

HATSE IMAGING

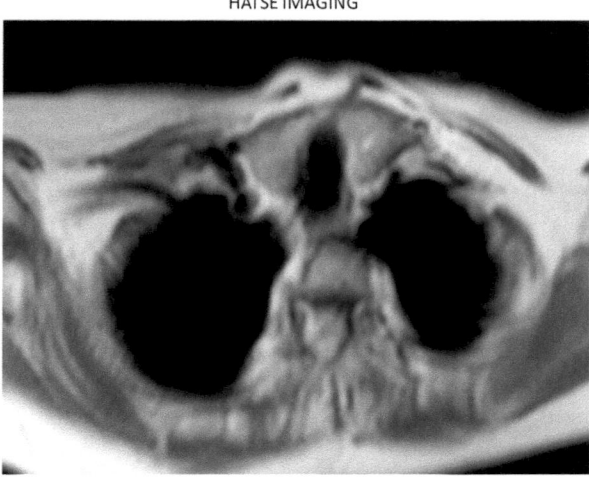

(A) Pulmonary embolism
(B) Aortic dissection
(C) Thyroid nodule
(D) Thymoma

The correct answer is C. The half-acquired turbo spin anatomical imaging demonstrates a heterogeneously enlarged thyroid gland with a possible nodule in the left lobe [12].

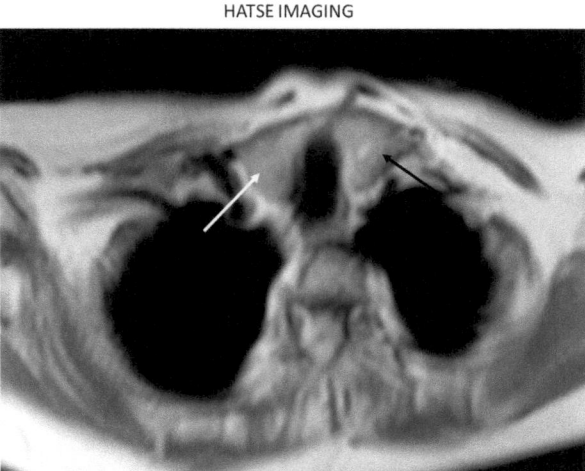

HATSE IMAGING

HATSE imaging demonstrates a heterogeneously, enlarged thyroid gland (white arrow) with a potential small nodule (black arrow).

111. What is the most likely diagnosis in the following images?

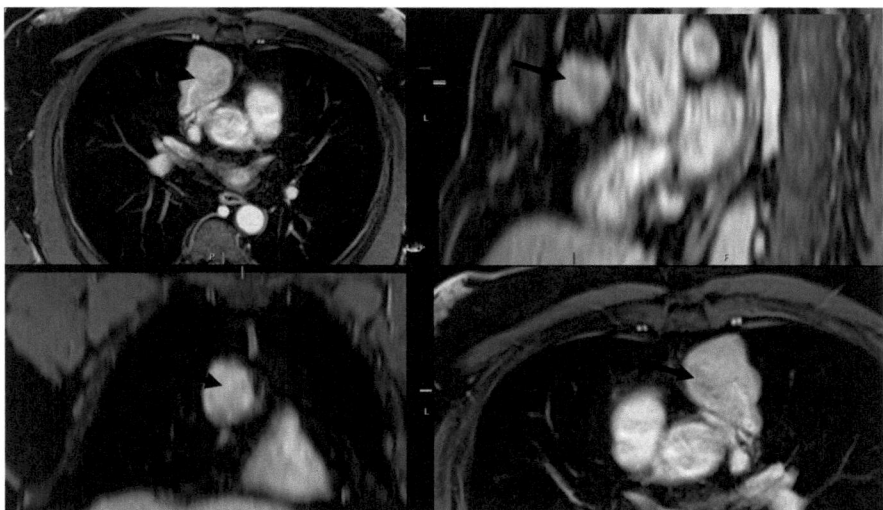

(A) Thymoma
(B) Aortic dissection
(C) Persistent left-sided supra vena cava
(D) Pericardial fat

The correct answer is A. An anterior mediastinal mass is located outside the pericardium [13]. The mass is well-circumscribed so unlikely to be pericardial fat. There is no aortic dissection seen. The most likely answer is a thymoma [14].

112. The following images demonstrate:

Coronal Scout Images

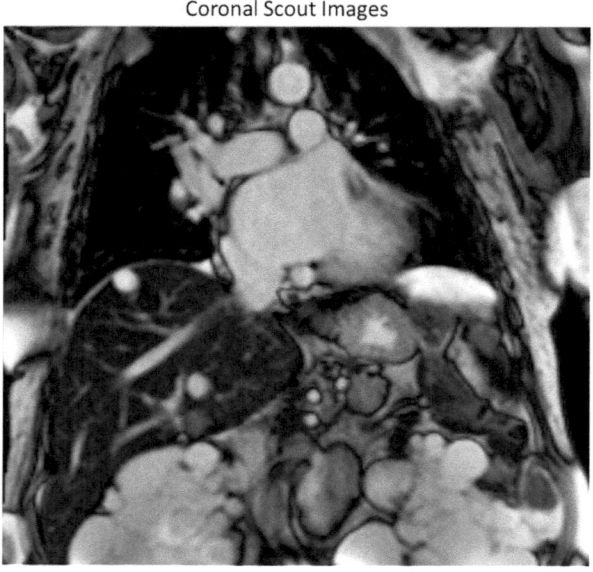

(A) Saddle pulmonary embolism
(B) Sinus venosus defect
(C) Lung mass
(D) Polycystic kidney/liver disease

The correct answer is D. The scout image demonstrates multiple hepatic and kidney cysts. This likely represents a diagnosis of polycystic kidney disease. Incidental findings occur commonly on scout images and need to be reported to referring providers, as major incidental findings can occur up to 12% of the time [15]. The most common organs are liver (16%), lung (15%), and kidney (14%). There is no clear lung mass demonstrated. We only see a glimpse of the left atrium, so not enough information to make a diagnosis of sinus venosus defect. We do not see any clot in the limited view of the pulmonary artery.

References

1. Kassem KM, Souka A, Harris DM, Parajuli S, Cook JL. Eosinophilic myocarditis: classic presentation of elusive disease. Circ Cardiovasc Imaging. 2019;12(9):e009487. https://doi.org/10.1161/CIRCIMAGING.119.009487.
2. Janus SE, Al-Kindi SG, Rashid I, Hoit BD. Cystic left ventricular mass: the utility of transthoracic echocardiography and cardiac MRI. BMJ Case Rep. 2021;14(2):e239985. https://doi.org/10.1136/bcr-2020-239985.
3. Chaosuwannakit N, Makarawate P. Left ventricular thrombi: insights from cardiac magnetic resonance imaging. Tomography. 2021;7(2):180–8. https://doi.org/10.3390/tomography7020016.
4. Srichai MB, Junor C, Rodriguez LL, Stillman AE, Grimm RA, Lieber ML, Weaver JA, Smedira NG, White RD. Clinical, imaging, and pathological characteristics of left ventricular thrombus: a comparison of contrast-enhanced magnetic resonance imaging, transthoracic echocardiography, and transesophageal echocardiography with surgical or pathological validation. Am Heart J. 2006;152(1):75–84. https://doi.org/10.1016/j.ahj.2005.08.021.
5. Duncan MD, Swinburne AJ, Sahni S, Zuckerman JE, Hacobian M. Small cell lung cancer presenting as a cardiac mass with embolic phenomena. Am J Med. 2017;130(2):e55–7. https://doi.org/10.1016/j.amjmed.2016.08.028.
6. Daye D, Ackman JB. Characterization of mediastinal masses by MRI: techniques and applications. Appl Radiol. 2017;10–22 https://doi.org/10.37549/AR2394.
7. Abbas A, Garfath-Cox KAG, Brown IW, Shambrook JS, Peebles CR, Harden SP. Cardiac MR assessment of cardiac myxomas. Br J Radiol. 2015;88(1045):20140599. https://doi.org/10.1259/bjr.20140599.
8. Chan AT, Dinsfriend W, Kim J, Yum B, Sultana R, Klebanoff CA, Plodkowski A, Perez Johnston R, Ginsberg MS, Liu J, Kim RJ, Steingart R, Weinsaft JW. Risk stratification of cardiac metastases using late gadolinium enhancement cardiovascular magnetic resonance: prognostic impact of hypo-enhancement evidenced tumor avascularity. J Cardiovasc Magn Reson. 2021;23(1):42. https://doi.org/10.1186/s12968-021-00727-2.
9. Motwani M, Kidambi A, Herzog BA, Uddin A, Greenwood JP, Plein S. MR imaging of cardiac tumors and masses: a review of methods and clinical applications. Radiology. 2013;268(1):26–43. https://doi.org/10.1148/radiol.13121239.
10. Bignotti B, Succio G, Nosenzo F, Perinetti M, Gristina L, Barbagallo S, Secondini L, Calabrese M, Tagliafico A. Breast findings incidentally detected on body MRI. SpringerPlus. 2016;5(1):781. https://doi.org/10.1186/s40064-016-2343-x.
11. Gibson LM, Paul L, Chappell FM, Macleod M, Whiteley WN, Salman RA-S, Wardlaw JM, Sudlow CLM. Potentially serious incidental findings on brain and body magnetic resonance imaging of apparently asymptomatic adults: systematic review and meta-analysis. BMJ. 2018;k4577 https://doi.org/10.1136/bmj.k4577.
12. Segal P. Incidental thyroid nodules detected on CT, MRI, or PET-CT scans correlate well with subsequent ultrasound evaluation; 2.
13. Chaturvedi A, Gange C, Sahin H, Chaturvedi A. Incremental value of magnetic resonance imaging in further characterizing hypodense mediastinal and paracardiac lesions identified on computed tomography. J Clin Imaging Sci. 2018;8:10. https://doi.org/10.4103/jcis.JCIS_63_17.
14. Grasso AE, O'Hanlon R, Locca D, Pennell DJ. Cardiovascular magnetic resonance of thymoma. Circulation. 2009;120(14):1453–5. https://doi.org/10.1161/CIRCULATIONAHA.108.830588.
15. Dunet V, Schwitter J, Meuli R, Beigelman-Aubry C. Incidental extracardiac findings on cardiac MR: systematic review and meta-analysis: IEFs on Cardiac MR Meta-Analysis. J Magn Reson Imaging. 2016;43(4):929–39. https://doi.org/10.1002/jmri.25053.

Chapter 8
Congenital

113. What is the congenital abnormality displayed below?

Steady state free precession imaging   HASTE Imaging

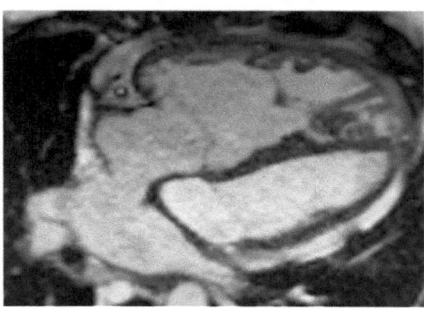 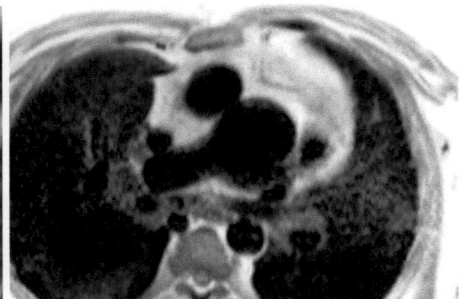

(A) D transposition of the great vessels with atrial switch
(B) L transposition of the great vessels with atrial switch
(C) D transposition of the great vessels with arterial switch
(D) L transposition of the great vessels with arterial switch

The correct answer is A. The patient has a D transposition of the great vessels with an atrial switch [1, 2].

© The Author(s), under exclusive license to Springer Nature
Switzerland AG 2023
S. G. Al-Kindi, S. E. Janus, *Cardiac MRI Certification Exam*,
https://doi.org/10.1007/978-3-031-25966-1_8

Steady state free precession imaging   HASTE Imaging

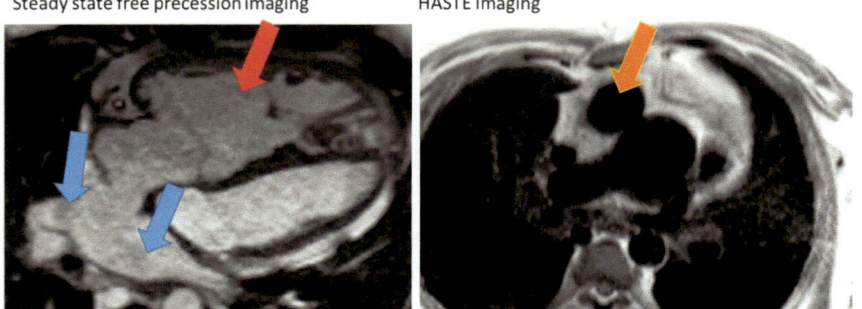

Steady state free precession imaging demonstrating baffle (blue arrows) connecting pulmonary veins to the right atrium and systemic right ventricle (red arrow). The aorta (orange arrow) can be seen arising from the right ventricle in the HASTE images. Therefore indicating a D transposition of great vessels with atrial switch procedure.

114. What is the congenital abnormality displayed below?

Steady state free precession imaging   HASTE Imaging

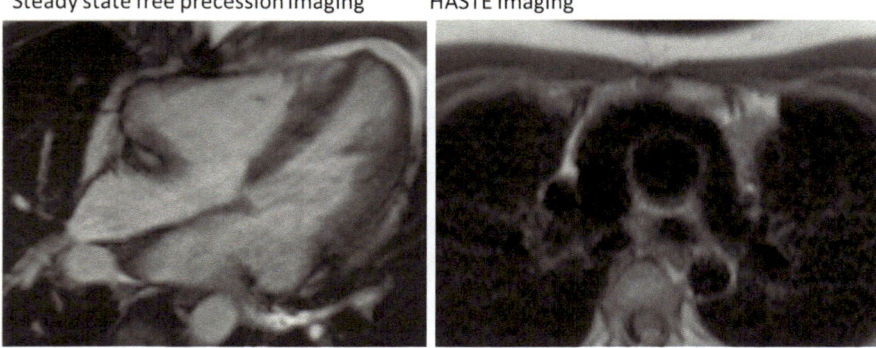

(A) D transposition of the great vessels with atrial switch
(B) L transposition of the great vessels with atrial switch
(C) D transposition of the great vessels with arterial switch
(D) L transposition of the great vessels with arterial switch

The correct answer is C. The images display the pulmonary artery arising from the morphologic right ventricle and straddling the aorta. This is seen in congenital D transposition with an arterial switch procedure [3].

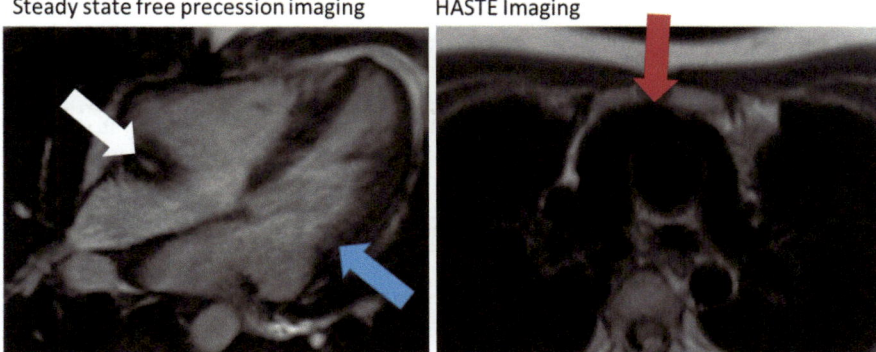

Steady state free precession imaging demonstrating normal right atrial to right ventricle connection (white arrow) and normal left atrium to left ventricle connection (blue arrow). The HASTE images demonstrate the pulmonary artery (red arrow) bifurcating around the aorta indicating a D transposition that has undergone an arterial switch.

115. Which of the following is *not* an indication to replace the pulmonary valve in a repair tetralogy of fallot patient?

(A) Severe pulmonary regurgitation with symptoms or decreased exercise tolerance
(B) Symptomatic, severe regurgitation with right ventricular dysfunction
(C) Asymptomatic patients with severe regurgitation with right ventricular dysfunction
(D) Asymptomatic severe pulmonic regurgitation with right ventricular systolic pressure 70 mmHg

The correct answer is D. Individuals with repaired tetralogy of fallot do not require repair for the regurgitation if the systolic pressure is only 70 mmHg, as the European society of cardiology recommends for pressure >80 mmHg or more when there is progressive tricuspid regurgitation. The remaining answers are all true based on the guidelines from Circulation 2014 [4].

Society	Class	Level of evidence	Indications for PVR
ACC/AHA	I	B	Severe regurgitation and symptoms and/or decreased exercise tolerance
	IIa	B	Severe pulmonary regurgitation combined with moderate to severe right ventricle dysfunction or moderate to severe right ventricle enlargement
		C	Severe PR and Symptomatic or sustained atrial or ventricular arrhythmias, moderate to severe TR
Canadian Cardiovascular Society	IIa	C	Progressive or moderate to severe right ventricular enlargement or ventricular arrhythmias or symptoms
European Society of Cardiology	I	C	Symptomatic patients with severe pulmonary stenosis or regurgitation
	IIa	C	Asymptomatic patients with severe pulmonary stenosis or regurgitation or decrease in exercise capacity, or progressive right ventricular dilation or dysfunction, progressive tricuspid regurgitation with right ventricle systolic pressure >80 mmHg, or sustained atrial/ventricular arrhythmias

116. What is demonstrated in the following image?

Steady State Free Precession

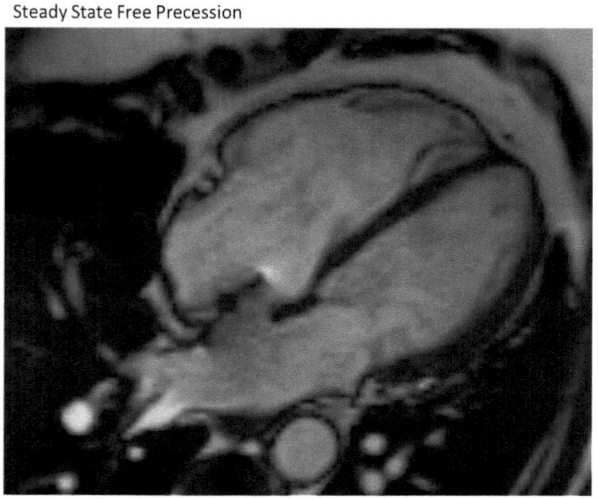

(A) Atrial septal defect
(B) Patent foramen ovale
(C) Ventricular septal defect
(D) Sinus venosus

The correct answer is A. There is a large secundum atrial septal defect present [5]. This orifice is too large for a patent foramen ovale that would appear more superiorly. A ventricular septal defect would be between the right and left ventricles. A sinus venosus defect would be much more superiorly located.

Steady State Free Precession

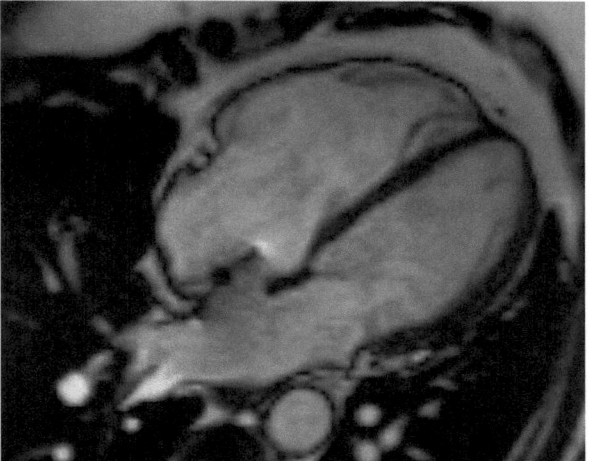

Steady State Free Precession- White arrows demonstrate large secundum atrial septal defect

117. What is the congenital abnormality displayed below?

Steady State Free Precession

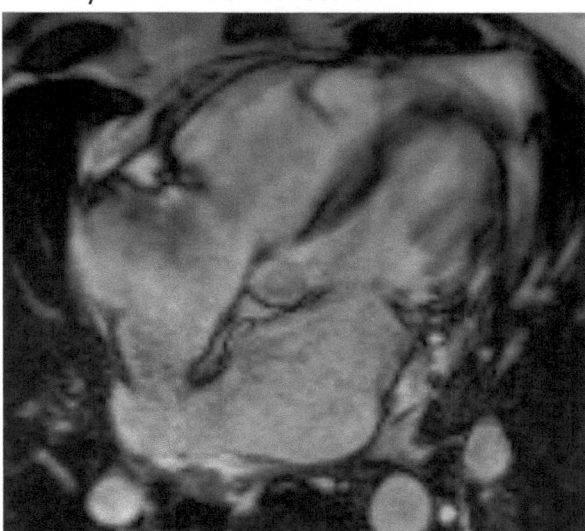

(A) Secundum atrial septal defect
(B) Primum atrial septal defect
(C) Sinus venosus defect
(D) Patent foramen ovale

The correct answer is C. Sinus venosus defect. The sinus venosus defect is an interatrial communication. Superior sinus venosus defects involve connection between the right upper pulmonary vein and superior vena cava. Inferior sinus venosus defect involves the inferior cava vein and the right lower pulmonary vein [6].

Steady State Free Precession

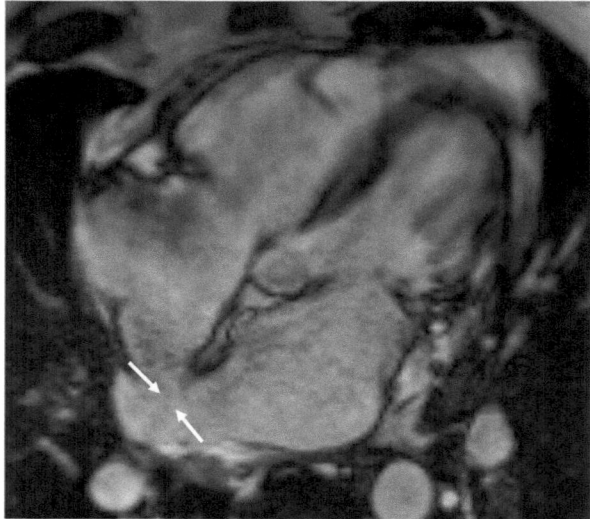

Steady State Free Precession- white arrows demonstrate a sinus venosus defect

118. What is the most likely diagnosis?

SSFP 4 Chamber

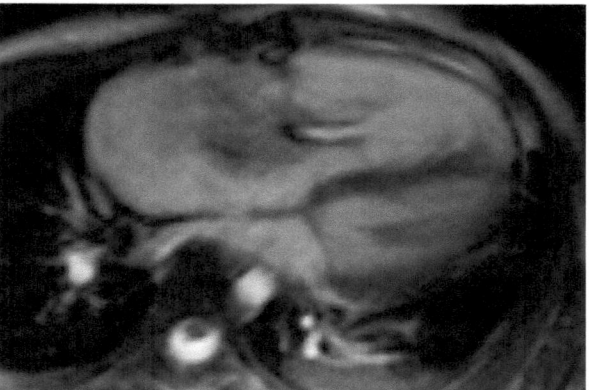

(A) Amyloid
(B) Myocarditis
(C) Ebstein's anomaly
(D) Non-compaction

The correct answer is C. Ebstein's anomaly. Ebstein's anomaly is a rare congenital disorder with apical displacement of the tricuspid valve [7]. The strict definition is >8 mm/m² of body surface area. The apical displacement leads to varying degrees of arterialization of the right ventricle. Myocarditis would be seen in T2 mapping and delayed enhancement imaging. Non-compaction will have a higher ratio of non-compacted to compacted myocardium. Amyloid cardiomyopathy typically presents with left ventricular hypertrophy and delayed enhancement.

119. What is the most likely diagnosis based on the images?

3D MRA Chest

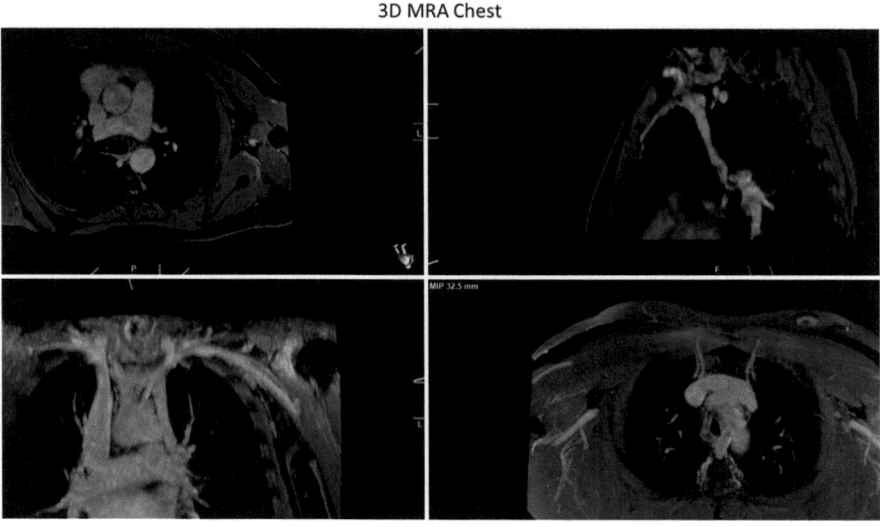

(A) Anomalous pulmonary venous return
(B) Supra vena cava thrombus
(C) Bovine Arch
(D) Ascending aortic aneurysm with combined dissection

The correct answer is A. The image demonstrates an abnormal connection of the left upper pulmonary vein connecting to the subclavian vein [8]. The supra vena cava does not demonstrate any thrombus. The aortic branch pattern is normal, but is not well visualized in the image above. There are no signs of aortic dissection on the axial stack.

3D MRA Chest

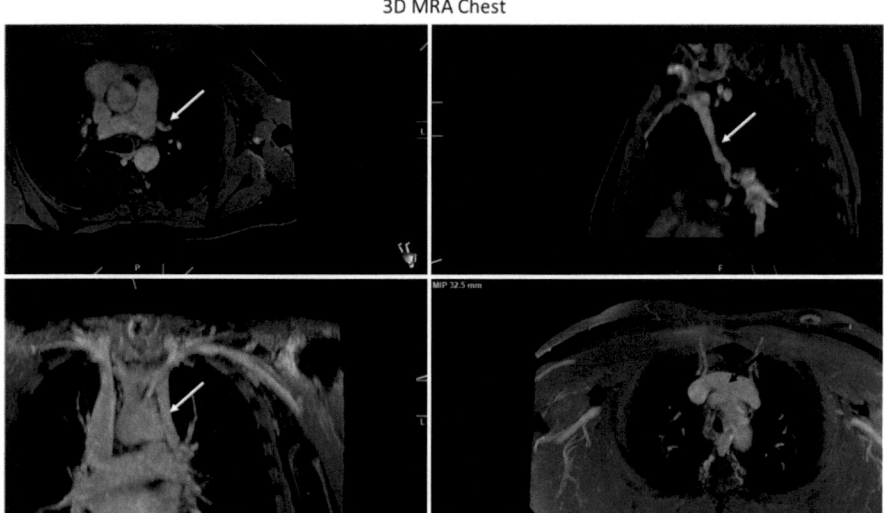

3D MRA Chest – demonstrating abnormal return of the left upper pulmonary vein (white arrow) to the subclavian vein (black arrow)

120. The most likely diagnosis is:

SSFP

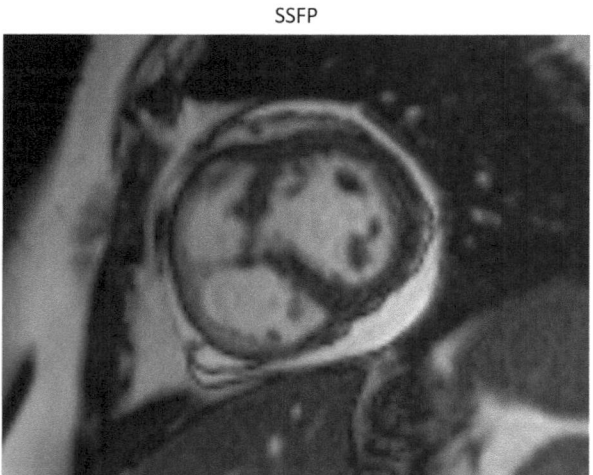

(A) Small membranous ventricular septal defect
(B) Small muscular ventricular septal defect
(C) Atrial septal defect
(D) Myocardial crypt

SSFP

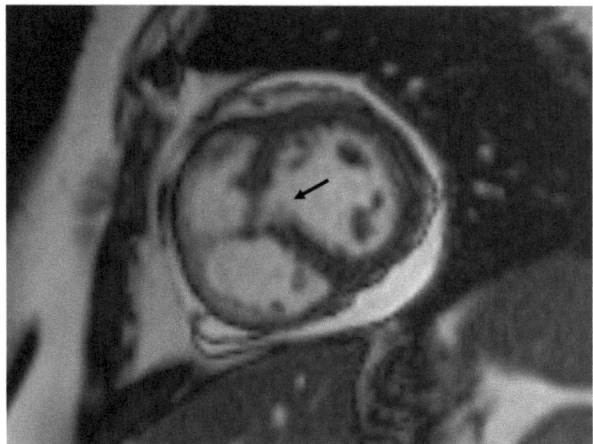

SSFP- demonstrating small, muscular ventricular septal
defect (black arrow)

The correct answer is B. The image demonstrates a muscular ventricular septal defect within the myocardium of the left ventricle [9]. A membranous defect would be more superior and better seen on the short axis of the aortic valve. An atrial septal defect would be seen between atrial chambers, this image demonstrates the left and right ventricles. The myocardial crypt is seen as a small indentation in the LV myocardium and is associated with hypertrophic cardiomyopathy.

121. What is the most likely diagnosis?

SSFP Short axis of Aortic Valve

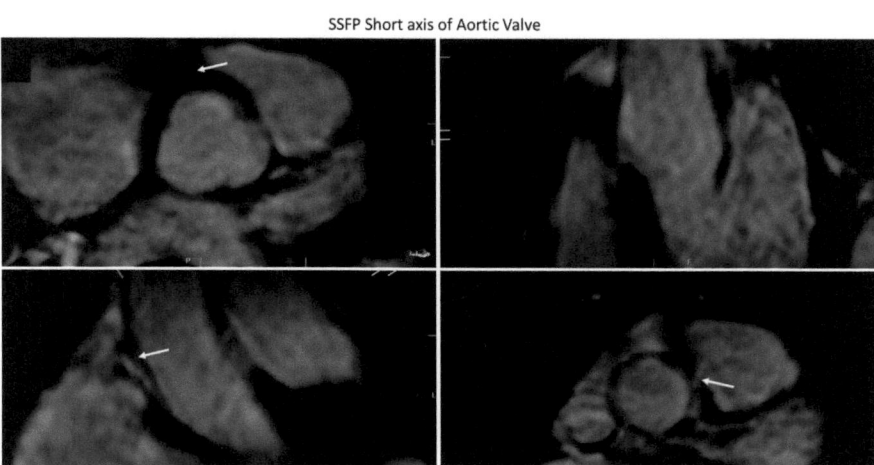

(A) Aortic stenosis
(B) Aortic dissection
(C) Aortic aneurysm
(D) Anomalous coronary origin

The correct answer is D. The short axis of the aortic valve demonstrates the right coronary originating from the left cusp with an inter-arterial (between pulmonary artery and aorta) and intra-arterial (courses into the pulmonary artery) course [10]. The valve is not well seen nor gradient provided to make a diagnosis of aortic stenosis. There is no acute aortic pathology to suggest dissection or aneurysm.

122. What is the most likely diagnosis?

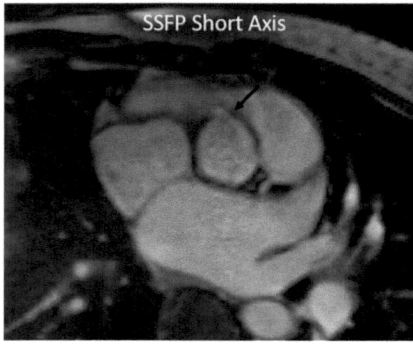 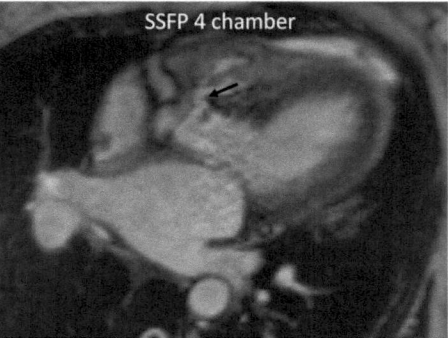

(A) Muscular ventricular septal defect
(B) Membranous ventricular septal defect
(C) Inlet ventricular septal defect
(D) Sinus of Valsalva aneurysm

The correct answer is B. The images demonstrate a short axis of the aortic valve showing a ventricular septal defect with communication into the right ventricle. The chamber demonstrates the defect in the membranous septum. A muscular ventricular septal defect would occur within the muscular portion and much more inferiorly in the left ventricle. An inlet ventricular septal defect would involve the atrioventricular canal. A sinus of Valsalva aneurysm would involve the aorta, not the left ventricle [11].

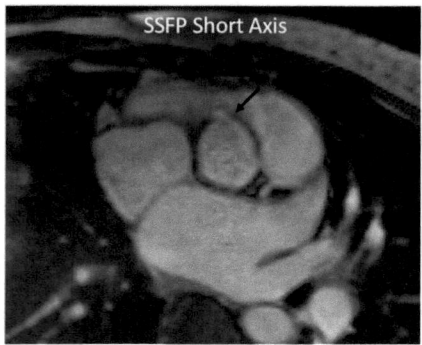 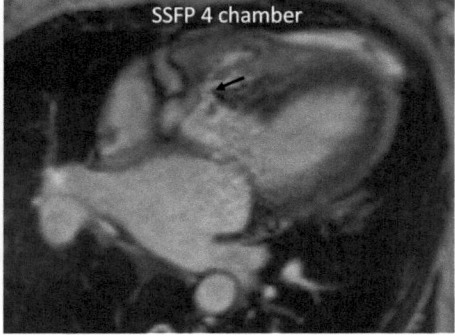

Black arrows demonstrating a membranous ventricular septal defect with communication between the left ventricle and the right ventricle.

123. What is the most likely diagnosis?

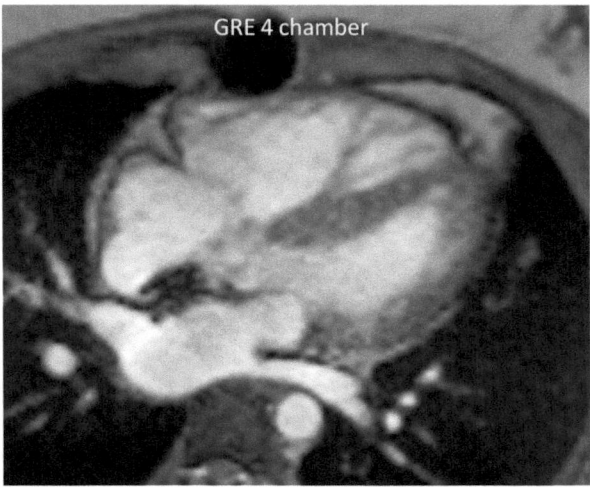

(A) Atrial septal defect with occluder device
(B) Myxoma
(C) Lipoma
(D) Clot in transit

The correct answer is A. The interatrial septum demonstrates a metallic structure with bilayered discs on each side of the interatrial septum. This is most consistent with an Atrial septal defect occluder device. A myxoma or lipoma would likely only be on one side of the interatrial septum. The consistency of the device with straight edges makes thrombus in transit less likely [12].

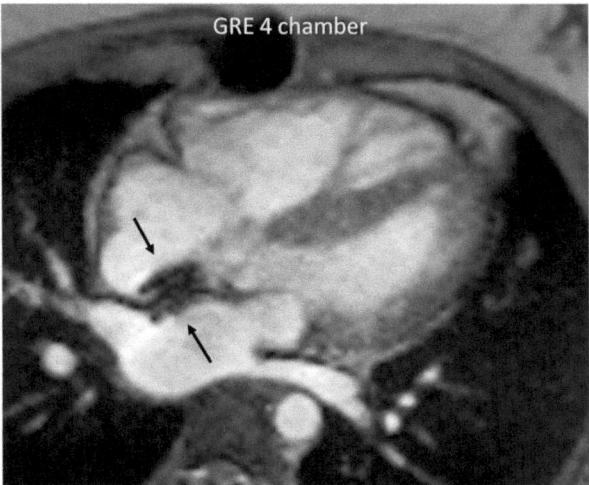

Black arrows demonstrating the occluder device with disks on each side of the intra-atrial septum.

124. What does the following image demonstrate?

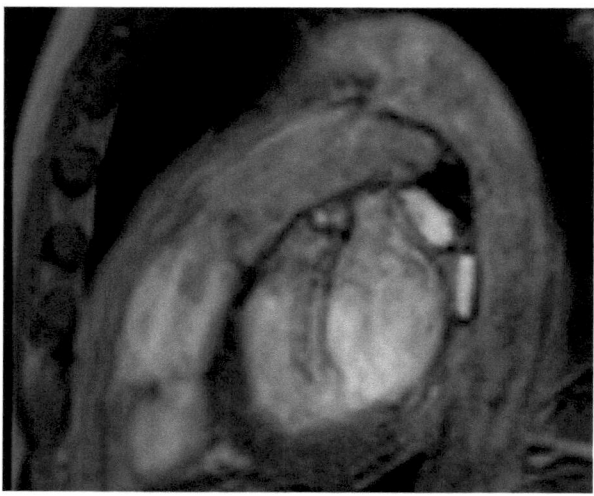

(A) Patent ductus arteriosus
(B) Pulmonary embolism in transit
(C) Aortic dissection
(D) Myocarditis

The correct answer is A. The image demonstrates a patent ductus arteriosus with a connection between the pulmonary artery and the aorta [11].

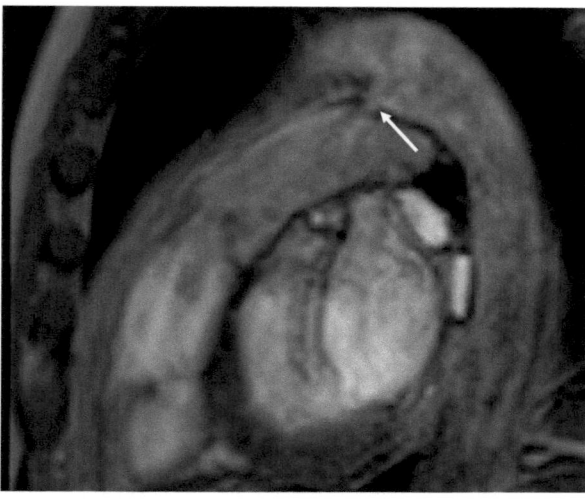

SSFP- demonstrates a connection between the aorta and pulmonary artery likely representing patent ductus arteriosus

125. What is the most likely diagnosis?

SSFP 4 chamber

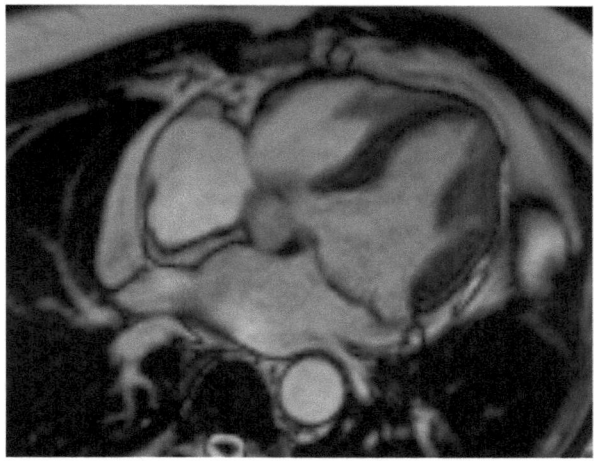

(A) Ebstein's anomaly
(B) Anomalous pulmonary venous return
(C) Ventricular septal defect
(D) Mitral annular disjunction

The correct answer is D. The mitral valve shows displacement. There is bileaflet mitral valve prolapse. The tricuspid is in the correct position, so not Ebstein's anomaly. There is evidence of anomalous pulmonary venous return. The ventricular septum appears to be intact [13].

SSFP 4 chamber

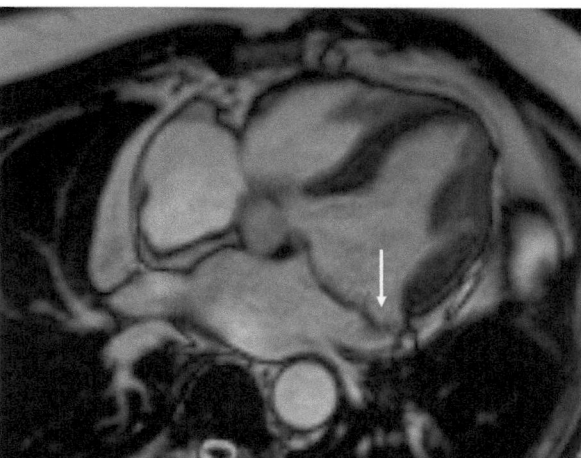

SSFP 4 chamber demonstrates displacement of the mitral valve (white arrow). This particular echo demonstrates Barlow's syndrome (mitral valve thickening, bileaflet mitral valve prolapse).

126. In what condition can the finding below be seen?

Delayed enhancement

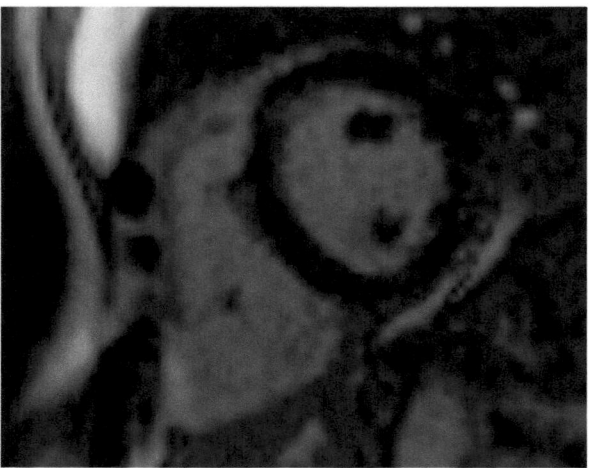

(A) LAD infarction
(B) Sarcoidosis
(C) Fabry's
(D) ARVC

Delayed enhancement

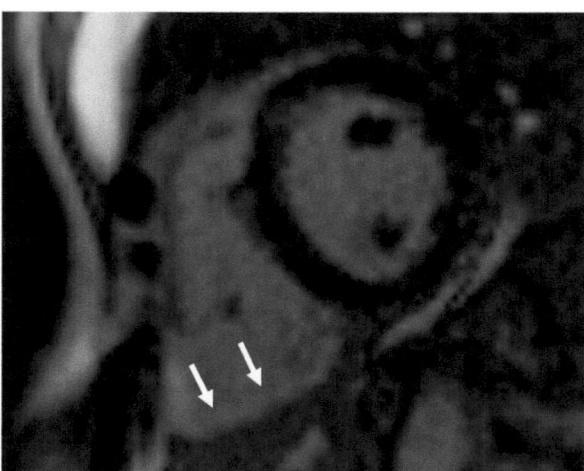

Delayed enhancement-
Demonstrating significant
enhancement in the right ventricle
(white arrows)

The correct answer is D. The image demonstrates fibrosis within the base of the right ventricle, which is most consistent with ARVC [14]. It is important to note, though, that RV LGE is not frequently seen in ARVC and is not a criterion for diagnosis. The presence of LGE can be supportive of the diagnosis, along with dyskinesis/akinesis and RV dilation/dysfunction. A LAD infarct would show fibrosis in the anterior wall. Sarcoidosis would show patchy fibrosis. Fabry's would show fatty infiltration in the right ventricle.

References

1. de Roos A. Role of cardiovascular magnetic resonance imaging in postoperative follow-up after the arterial switch operation for transposition of the great arteries. Circ Cardiovasc Imaging. 2016;9(9):e005463. https://doi.org/10.1161/CIRCIMAGING.116.005463.
2. Ntsinjana HN, Hughes ML, Taylor AM. The role of cardiovascular magnetic resonance in pediatric congenital heart disease. J Cardiovasc Magn Reson. 2011;13(1):51. https://doi.org/10.1186/1532-429X-13-51.
3. Chelliah A, Shah AM, Farooqi KM, Einstein AJ, Han BK. Cardiovascular CT in cyanotic congenital heart disease. Curr Cardiovasc Imaging Rep. 2019;12(7):30. https://doi.org/10.1007/s12410-019-9507-3.
4. Weinberg CR, McElhinney DB. Pulmonary valve replacement in tetralogy of Fallot. Circulation. 2014;130(9):795–8. https://doi.org/10.1161/CIRCULATIONAHA.114.005551.
5. Holmvang G, Palacios IF, Vlahakes GJ, Dinsmore RE, Miller SW, Liberthson RR, Block PC, Ballen B, Brady TJ, Kantor HL. Imaging and sizing of atrial septal defects by magnetic resonance. Circulation. 1995;92(12):3473–80. https://doi.org/10.1161/01.CIR.92.12.3473.
6. Schantz D, Thompson D, Warren A. Magnetic resonance imaging-aided diagnosis of an inferior sinus venosus defect: a case report. Pediatr Cardiol. 2010;31(4):564–6. https://doi.org/10.1007/s00246-010-9643-7.
7. Attenhofer Jost CH, Connolly HM, Dearani JA, Edwards WD, Danielson GK. Ebstein's anomaly. Circulation. 2007;115(2):277–85. https://doi.org/10.1161/CIRCULATIONAHA.106.619338.
8. Robinson BL, Kwong RY, Varma PK, Wolfe M, Couper G. Magnetic resonance imaging of complex partial anomalous pulmonary venous return in adults. Circulation. 2014;129(1) https://doi.org/10.1161/CIRCULATIONAHA.113.005004.
9. Secchi F, Giardino A, Fabiano S, Fesslova V, Sardanelli F. Visualization of a small ventricular septal defect at first-pass contrast-enhanced cardiac magnetic resonance imaging. J Clin Imaging Sci. 2013;3:59. https://doi.org/10.4103/2156-7514.124083.
10. Lee H-J, Hong YJ, Kim HY, Lee J, Hur J, Choi BW, Chang H-J, Nam JE, Choe KO, Kim YJ. Anomalous origin of the right coronary artery from the left coronary sinus with an inter-arterial course: subtypes and clinical importance. Radiology. 2012;262(1):101–8. https://doi.org/10.1148/radiol.11110823.
11. Wang ZJ, Reddy GP, Gotway MB, Yeh BM, Higgins CB. Cardiovascular shunts: MR imaging evaluation. RadioGraphics. 2003;23(Suppl 1):S181–94. https://doi.org/10.1148/rg.23si035503.
12. Roy D, Sharma R, Bunce N, Ward D, Brecker S. Selecting the optimal closure device in patients with atrial septal defects and patent foramen ovale. Interv Cardiol. 2012;4(1):85–100. https://doi.org/10.2217/ica.11.90.

13. Perazzolo Marra M, Basso C, De Lazzari M, Rizzo S, Cipriani A, Giorgi B, Lacognata C, Rigato I, Migliore F, Pilichou K, Cacciavillani L, Bertaglia E, Frigo AC, Bauce B, Corrado D, Thiene G, Iliceto S. Morphofunctional abnormalities of mitral annulus and arrhythmic mitral valve prolapse. Circ Cardiovasc Imaging. 2016;9(8) https://doi.org/10.1161/CIRCIMAGING.116.005030.
14. Liu Y, Yu J, Liu J, Wu B, Cui Q, Shen W, Xia S. Prognostic value of late gadolinium enhancement in arrhythmogenic right ventricular cardiomyopathy: a meta-analysis. Clin Radiol. 2021;76(8):628.e9–628.e15. https://doi.org/10.1016/j.crad.2021.04.002.

Chapter 9
Magnetic Resonance Angiography

127. What do the following MRA images likely represent?

Haste imaging   T1 Inphase MRA

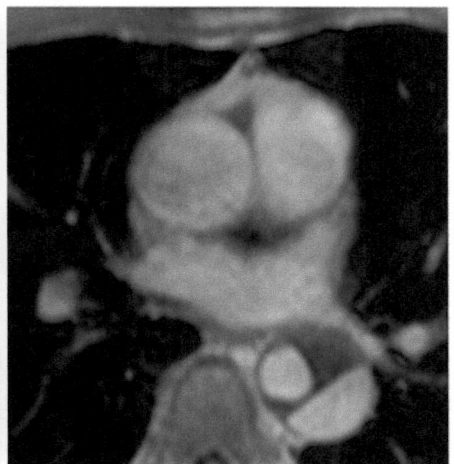

(A) Stanford type A aortic dissection
(B) Stanford type B aortic dissection
(C) Penetrating ulcer
(D) Pulmonary embolism

The correct answer is B. The descending aorta demonstrates a dissection with a larger false lumen [1]. There is no evidence on the image of a penetrating ulcer. While not visualized well, the pulmonary arteries do not demonstrate a pulmonary embolism.

© The Author(s), under exclusive license to Springer Nature Switzerland AG 2023
S. G. Al-Kindi, S. E. Janus, *Cardiac MRI Certification Exam*,
https://doi.org/10.1007/978-3-031-25966-1_9

Haste imaging   MRA

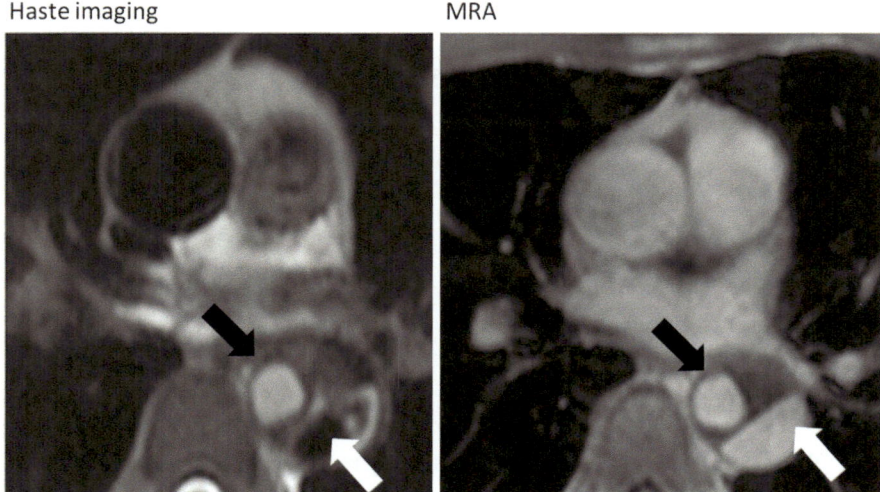

Haste imaging demonstrating the false lumen (white arrow) and the true lumen (black arrow).

128. In an individual with coarctation of the aorta, which of the following should be true regarding volume flow if there are collaterals present?

MRA

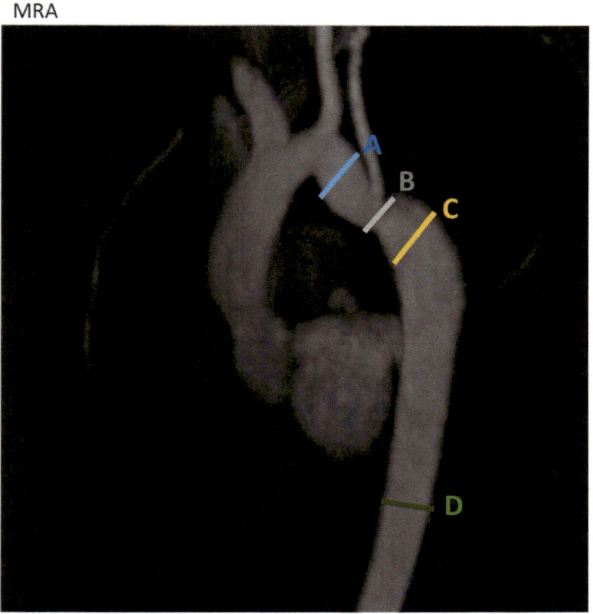

(A) A>D
(B) A>B
(C) D>A
(D) D>C

The correct answer is C. The flow in the distal aorta should be greater than the ascending aorta. Due to significant branch collaterals feeding blood to the periphery, increased flow volume will be present in the descending if there are indeed significant collaterals [2]. Therefore, D being greater than the proximal ascending aorta makes the most likely diagnosis of significant coarctation.

129. When measuring aortic diameters on MRA, what is the considered standard technique?

(A) Inner edge to inner edge
(B) Inner edge to outer edge
(C) Outer edge to inner edge
(D) Outer edge to outer edger

The correct answer is A. The recommendation is to measure the inner edge to inner edge when measuring the aorta [3].

130. What does the following MRA demonstrate?

MRA

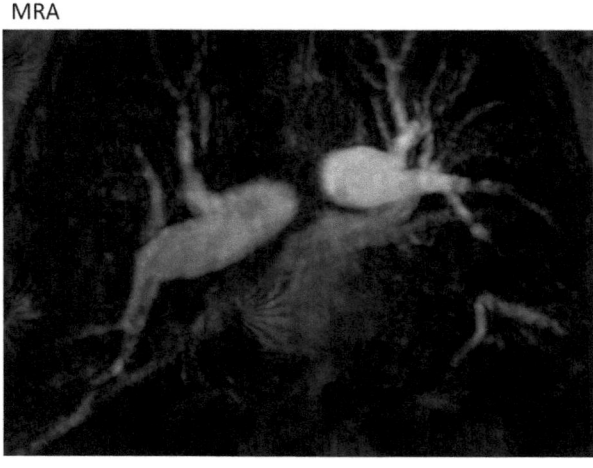

(A) Anomalous pulmonary artery return
(B) Anomalous pulmonary vein return
(C) Pulmonary artery embolism
(D) Tetralogy of fallot

The correct answer is C. The image demonstrates a sub-segmental pulmonary embolism. There is no definitive evidence of anomalous return or tetralogy of fallot.

MRA

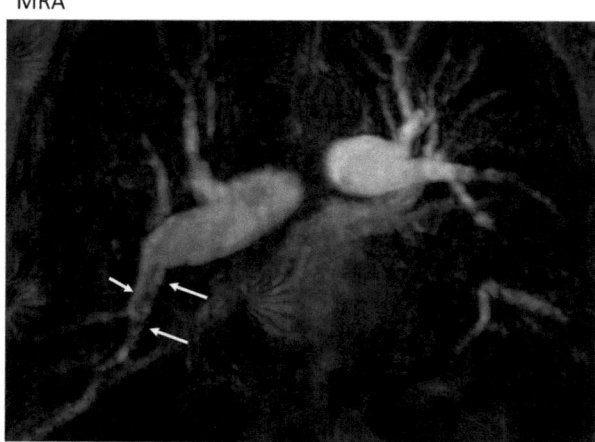

MRA- with pulmonary angiogram demonstrating
subsegmental pulmonary embolism (white arrows)

131. Which of the following is not an indication of peripheral MRA?

(A) Leg weakness
(B) Intermittent claudication, worse with exertion
(C) Planned revascularization of limb ischemia
(D) Following for endovascular leak of graft material

The correct answer is A. Leg weakness is a neurologic sign. Claudication, planned revascularization and following for endovascular leak of a graft are all indications for MRA [4].

132. Which of the following sequences involve contrast MRA?

(A) QISS
(B) TWIST
(C) CEST
(D) A, B, and C
(E) B and C

The correct answer is E. TWIST, CEST, and bolus chase are all series that involve gadolinium-enhanced MRA. QISS is a non-gadolinium-based series [5].

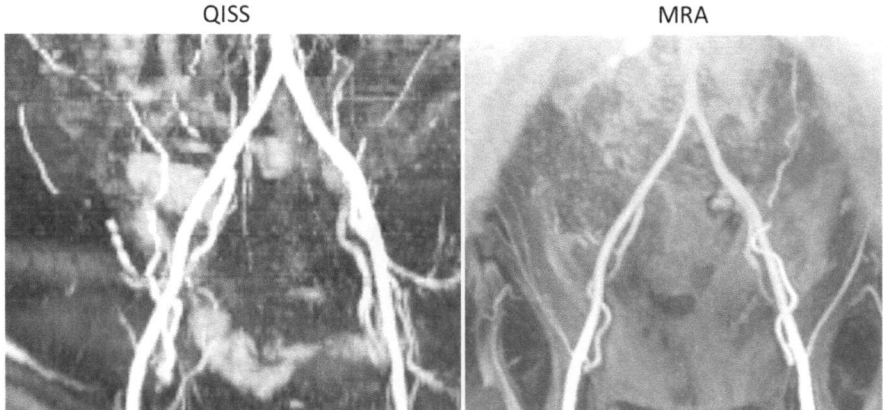

133. Which of the following is true?

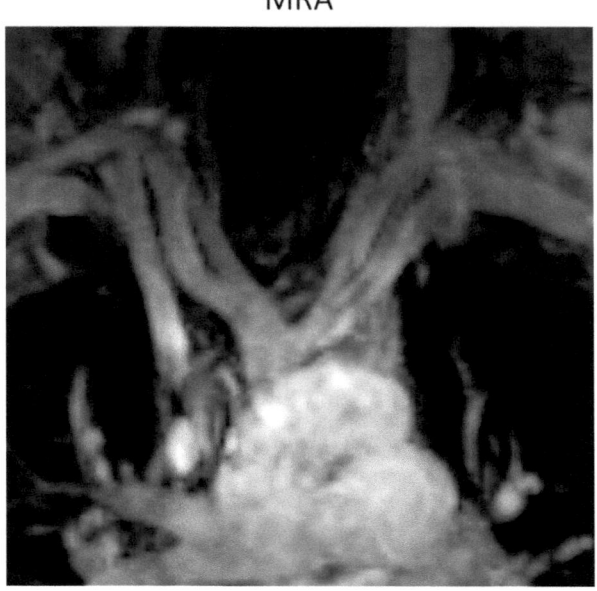

(A) The MRA demonstrates bovine arch
(B) The MRA demonstrates aortic dissection
(C) The MRA demonstrates pulmonary embolism
(D) The MRA demonstrates anomalous pulmonary venous return

The correct answer is A. The MRA demonstrates the left common carotid and the left subclavian branching from a common trunk making this a bovine arch [6]. There is no clear aortic dissection or pulmonary embolism seen. The pulmonary venous return is not well demonstrated to make a diagnosis of anomalous pulmonary venous return.

MRA

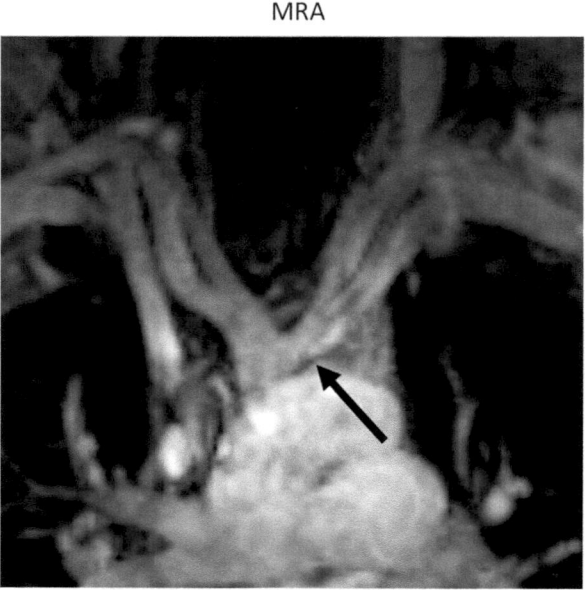

MRA- demonstrate a bovine arch with
the left common carotid originating
along with the left subclavian from a

134. What is the most likely diagnosis based on the images below?

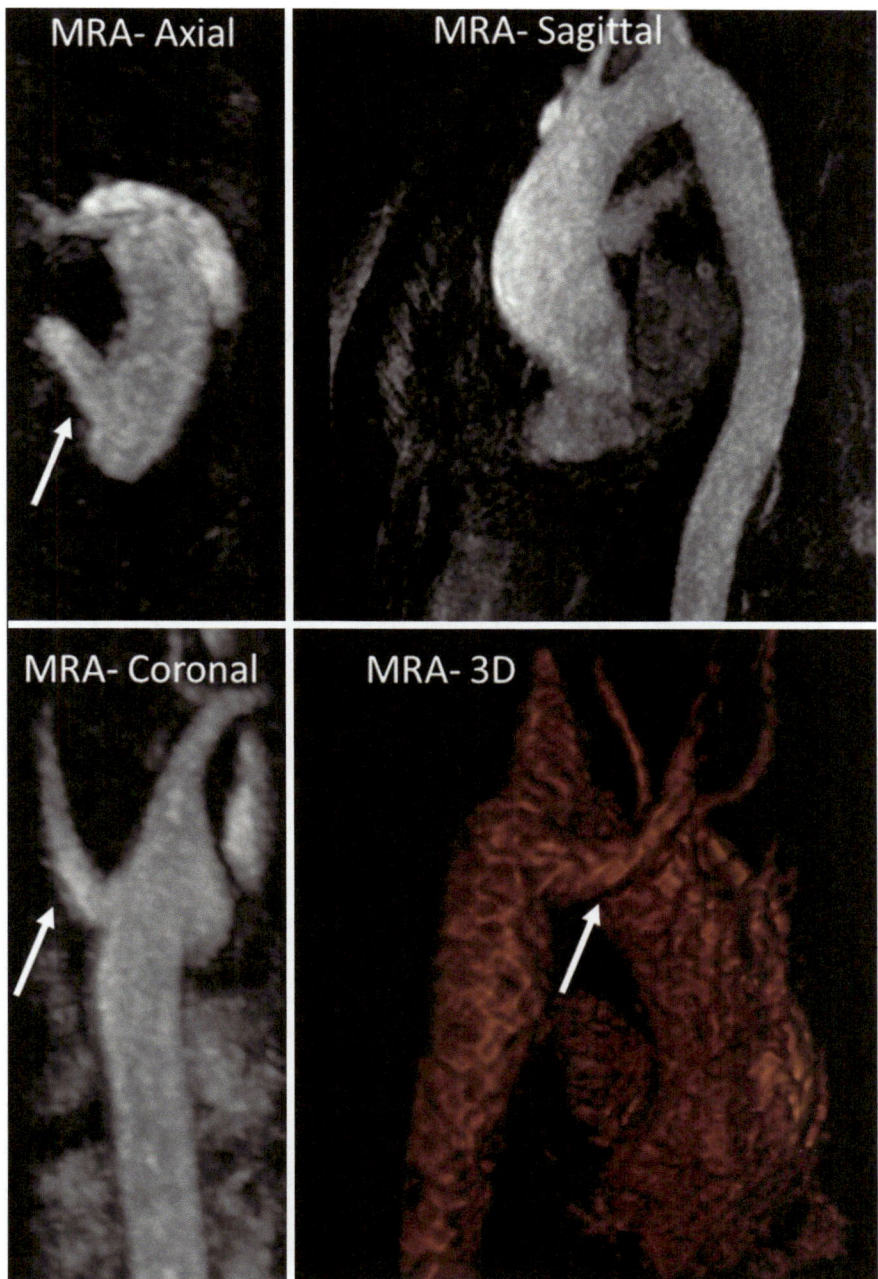

(A) Aberrant right subclavian
(B) Aortic intramural hematoma
(C) Carotid artery stenosis
(D) Clot in transit

The correct answer is A. The MRA demonstrates an aberrant right subclavian artery with a retro esophageal course. An aberrant right subclavian running posterior to the esophagus can cause dysphagia. There is no dissection noted in the aorta. The carotids do not demonstrate any stenosis. There is no clot in transit seen [7].

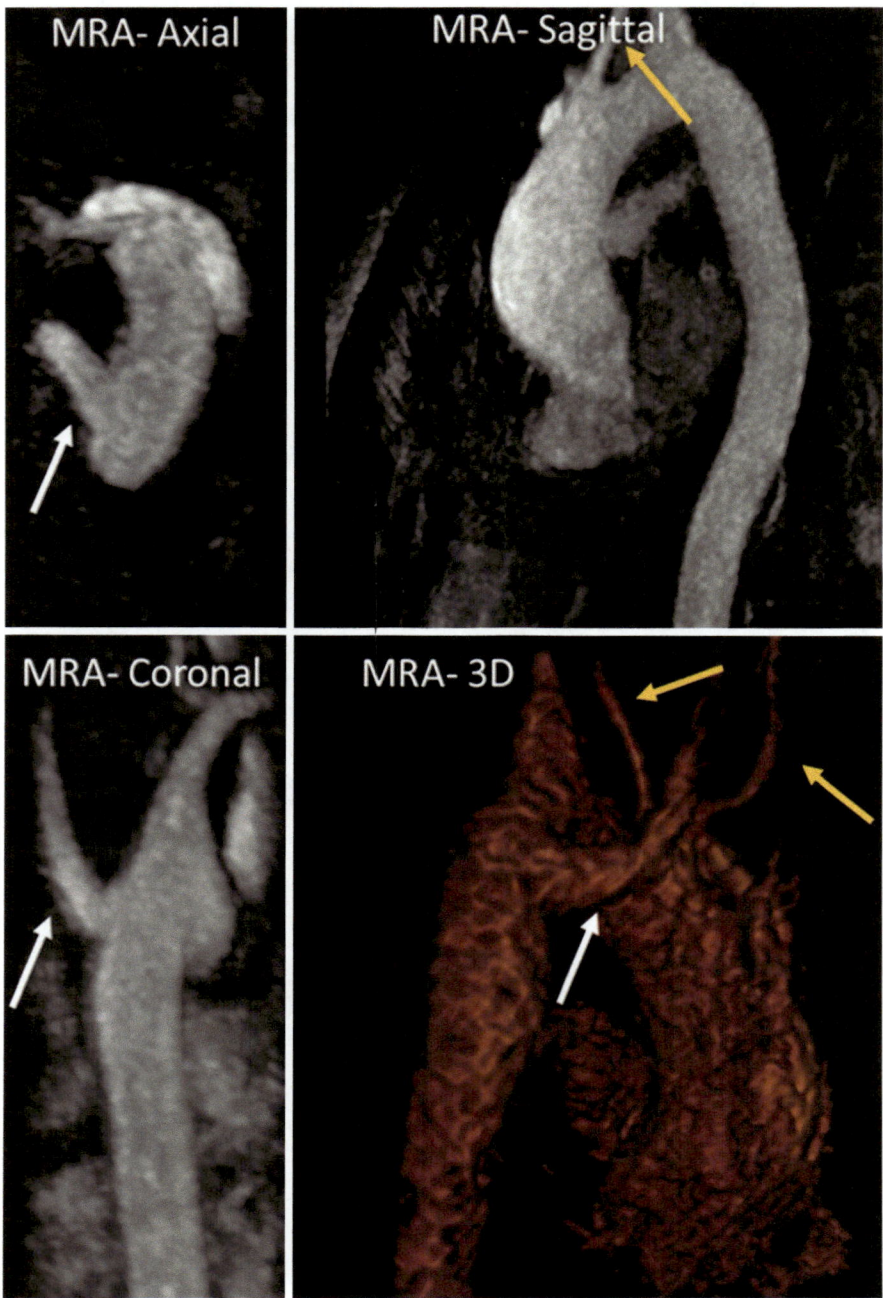

135. What is the most likely diagnosis?

SSFP

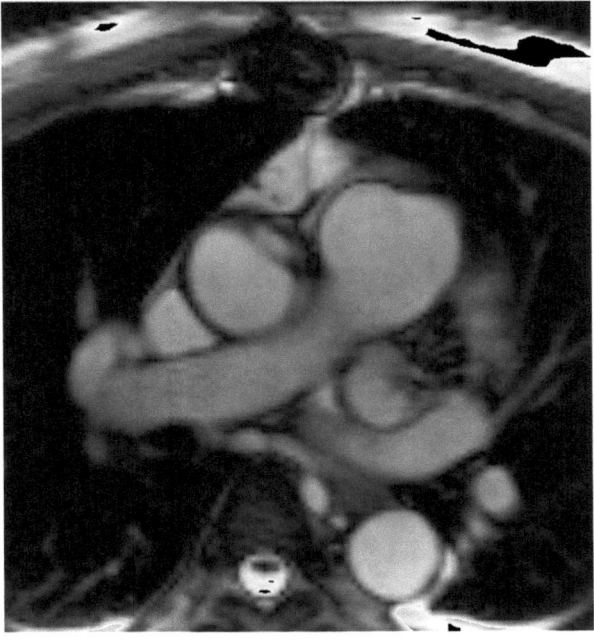

(A) L Transposition of the great vessels
(B) D Transposition of the great vessels
(C) Stanford type A dissection
(D) Stanford type B dissection

The correct answer is C. The image demonstrates a possible flap in the ascending aorta with a false lumen. This is concerning for a Stanford type A dissection. There is no evidence of L or D transposition of the great vessels as the pulmonary artery is anterior to the aorta. The descending aorta does not demonstrate any dissection flap. SSFp is an excellent series to identify and determine true vs false lumen as is HASTE imaging [8].

SSFP

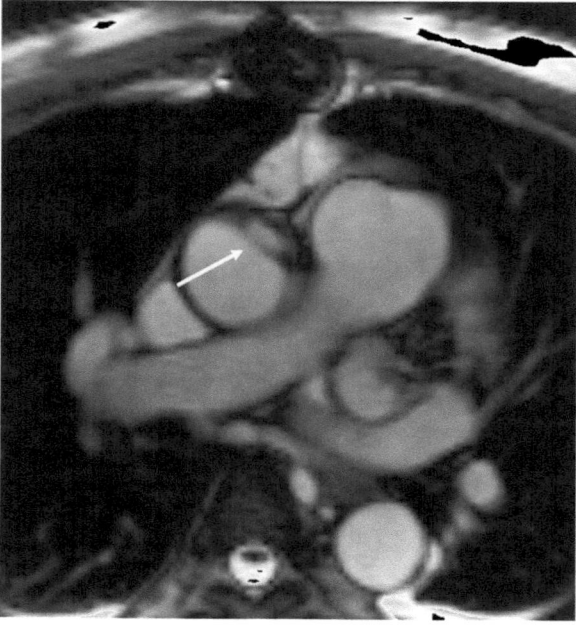

SSFP Imaging demonstrating a flap in the aorta
likely representing aortic dissection (white
arrow)

136. What is the most likely diagnosis?

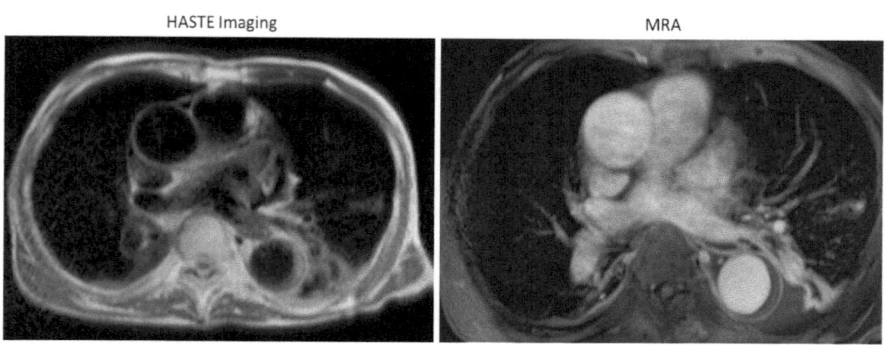

(A) Aortic intramural hematoma
(B) Pulmonary embolism
(C) Anomalous pulmonary venous return
(D) Penetrating ulcer

The correct answer is A. The descending thoracic aorta demonstrates a crescent-shaped intramural hematoma. The smooth filling defect in the descending aorta likely represents an intramural hematoma. There is no evidence of pulmonary embolism in the pulmonary artery. We do not clearly see pulmonary veins to comment on abnormal returns. The smooth shape appears more likely a hematoma than penetrating ulcer.

137. The following images demonstrate:

HASTE   STIR

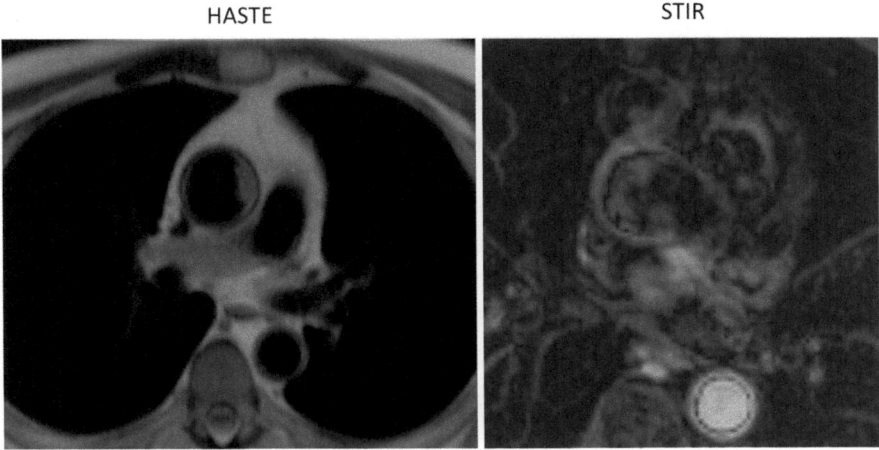

(A) Aortic dissection
(B) Aortic penetrating ulcer
(C) Aortitis
(D) Pulmonary embolism

The correct answer is C. This is HASTE imaging of an individual with giant cell arteritis who had concomitant aortic involvement. There is a thickening in the ascending and descending aorta. STIR imaging demonstrates severe inflammation within the descending aorta especially [9].

HASTE   STIR

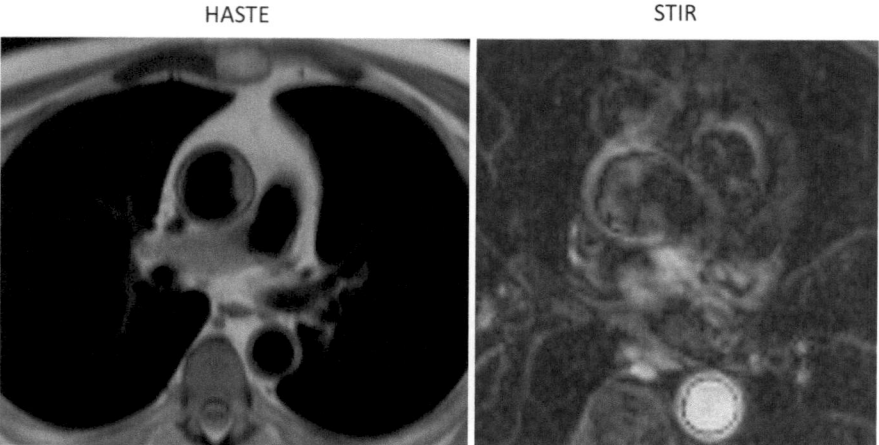

HASTE imaging demonstrating thickened aorta. STIR imaging demonstrating aortic inflammation

138. What is the likely diagnosis on the following images in a 54-year-old prior to ascending aortic aneurysm who underwent replacement with gel-weave graft?

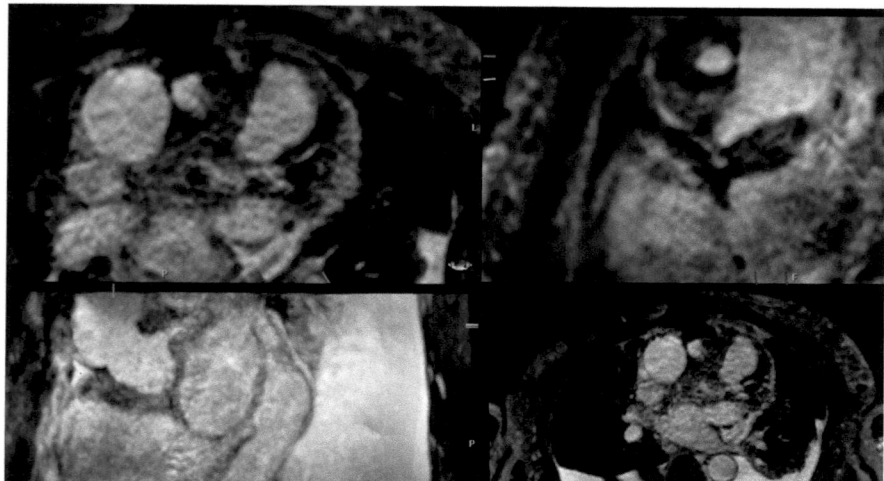

(A) Ascending aortic dissection
(B) Intramural hematoma
(C) Descending thoracic aortic dissection
(D) Endoleak

The correct answer is D. The images demonstrate an endoleak through the ascending aortic graft [10]. There is no intimate so unlikely another ascending aortic dissection. There are no signs of an intramural hematoma. The limited shots of the descending aorta do not show dissection.

MRA

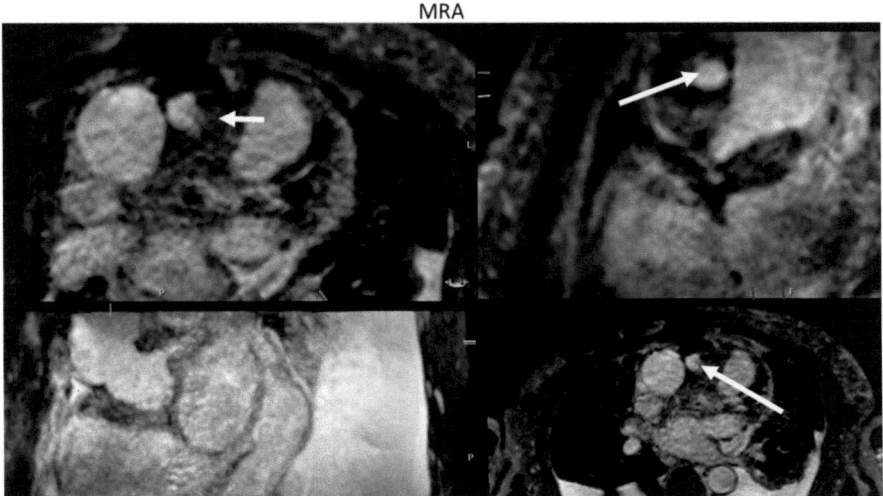

MRA demonstrating endo leak type III graft failure. There is a sac of fluid which is communicating with the aorta which represents an endoleak.

References

1. Armerding MD, Rubin GD, Beaulieu CF, Slonim SM, Olcott EW, Samuels SL, Jorgensen MJ, Semba CP, Jeffrey RB, Dake MD. Aortic aneurysmal disease: assessment of Stent-Graft treatment—CT versus conventional angiography. Radiology. 2000;215(1):138–46. https://doi.org/10.1148/radiology.215.1.r00ap28138.
2. Nguyen L, Cook SC. Coarctation of the aorta. Cardiol Clin. 2015;33(4):521–30. https://doi.org/10.1016/j.ccl.2015.07.011.
3. Hout M. How to measure the aorta using MRI: a practical guide. JMRI-ISMRM Recomm 971. 2020.
4. Chaikof EL, Dalman RL, Eskandari MK, Jackson BM, Lee WA, Mansour MA, Mastracci TM, Mell M, Murad MH, Nguyen LL, Oderich GS, Patel MS, Schermerhorn ML, Starnes BW. The Society for Vascular Surgery practice guidelines on the care of patients with an abdominal aortic aneurysm. J Vasc Surg. 2018;67(1):2–77.e2. https://doi.org/10.1016/j.jvs.2017.10.044.
5. Elster A. Phase-contrast MRA. In: MRI quest. https://mriquestions.com/phase-contrast-mra.html. Accessed 10 Jun 2022.
6. Layton KF, Kallmes DF, Cloft HJ, Lindell EP, Cox VS. Bovine aortic arch variant in humans: clarification of a common misnomer. Am J Neuroradiol 9.
7. Gonzalo C, Marjani M. Dysphagia Lusoria caused by an aberrant right subclavian artery. Korean J Gastroenterol. 2022;79(3):135–7. https://doi.org/10.4166/kjg.2022.037.

8. Weigang E, Nienaber CA, Rehders TC, Ince H, Vahl C-F, Beyersdorf F. Management of patients with aortic dissection. Dtsch Ärztebl Int. 2008. https://doi.org/10.3238/arztebl.2008.0639
9. Restrepo CS, Ocazionez D, Suri R, Vargas D. Aortitis: imaging spectrum of the infectious and inflammatory conditions of the aorta. RadioGraphics. 2011;31(2):435–51. https://doi.org/10.1148/rg.312105069.
10. van der Laan MJ, Bakker CJG, Blankensteijn JD, Bartels LW. Dynamic CE-MRA for Endoleak classification after endovascular aneurysm repair. Eur J Vasc Endovasc Surg. 2006;31(2):130–5. https://doi.org/10.1016/j.ejvs.2005.08.014.

Chapter 10
Flow Quantification

139. To become more sensitive to small flow quantities, what should you do to the velocity encoding?

(A) Increase TR
(B) Increase the velocity (VENC)
(C) Decrease the velocity (VENC)
(D) Decrease the flip angle

The correct answer is C. By decreasing the VENC, you will become more sensitive to low flow quantities like atrial septal defects or patent foramen ovale [1]. If you do not change the velocity, you will not become more or less sensitive. Higher velocity encoding prevents aliasing of the velocity.

© The Author(s), under exclusive license to Springer Nature Switzerland AG 2023
S. G. Al-Kindi, S. E. Janus, *Cardiac MRI Certification Exam*,
https://doi.org/10.1007/978-3-031-25966-1_10

140. Name the most likely diagnosis.

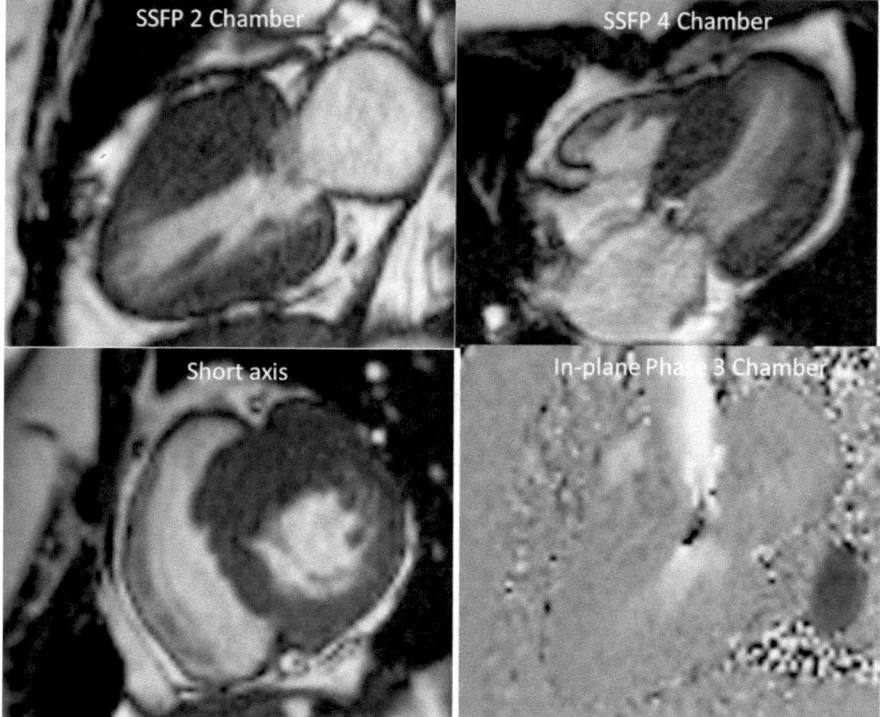

(A) Systolic anterior motion
(B) Mitral regurgitation
(C) Amyloid
(D) Myocarditis

The correct answer is A. The in-plane flow demonstrates systolic anterior motion of the mitral in the LVOT [2]. This is consistent with SAM from hypertrophic cardiomyopathy. The septum is thickened by >3 cm. While there may be some mitral regurgitation in the four chamber, the in-plane flow is demonstrating an outflow tract gradient. While amyloid can cause hypertrophy, the asymmetric hypertrophy and degree of hypertrophy make hypertrophic cardiomyopathy much more likely.

141. Which of the following is false?

(A) Slower-moving protons undergo less phase shift than faster-moving protons
(B) Through plane velocity encoding can provide quantification of flow
(C) The magnitude image contains directionally sensitive measurements
(D) It involves an equal and opposite phase shift

The correct answer is C. The remaining answers are all true. Slower-moving protons have less phase shift than faster-moving protons. Through plane encoding provides quantification of the flow. The phase shift is equal and opposite [3]. The only answer that is false is the magnitude image does not contain useful directionally sensitive measurements. The magnitude images are directionally insensitive.

Velocity Encoding

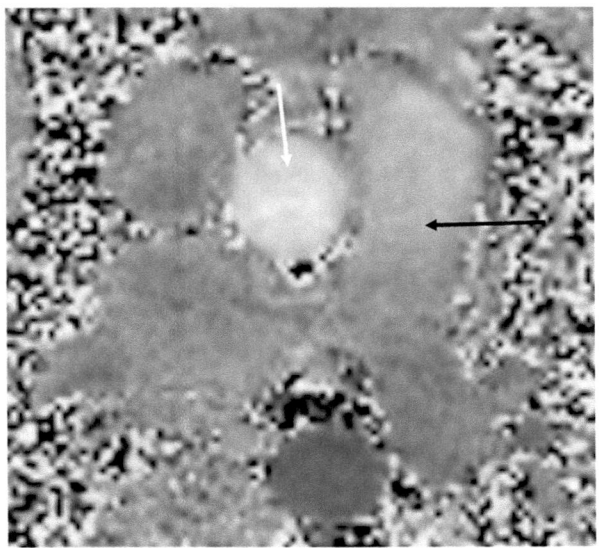

Velocity Encoding- White arrow (aorta) demonstrating through plane velocity encoding which can quantify flow. Black arrow (pulmonary artery) demonstrating in plane flow encoding, qualitative.

142. To velocity encode, one uses:

(A) Unipolar gradients
(B) Bipolar gradients
(C) Tripolar gradients
(D) Gadolinium-enhanced imaging

The correct answer is B. In order to obtain phase encoding, bipolar gradients are placed along the cardinal direction (x, y, and z axes) and measure the phase shift of the proton flow [3].

143. It is possible to display velocity phase-encoded images as all of the following except:

(A) Directionally insensitive
(B) Directionally sensitive color scale
(C) Directionally sensitive gray scale
(D) All of the above are true.

The correct answer is D. Velocity encoding can be displayed as directionally insensitive, directionally sensitive in both color and gray scale [4].

144. Which of the following is true?

(A) Cardiac output can be calculated via phase encoding
(B) Cardiac output can be calculated via myocardial tracing
(C) Both A and B
(D) Neither A nor B

The correct answer is C. Cardiac output can be calculated by either phase encoding or myocardial tracing [1].

145. What is the starting velocity for the aortic and pulmonic valves?

(A) 150 cm/s and 100 cm/s
(B) 200 cm/s and 100 cm/s
(C) 100 cm/s and 50 cm/s
(D) 50 cm/s and 50 cm/s

The correct answer is A. Most books cite initial velocity as 150–200 cm/s for aortic valve [5] and 100 cm/s for the pulmonic [6]. While some patients will alias at this low velocity, regurgitant volume will be more accurately calculated when the velocity is set slightly lower [7]. An initial velocity of 200 cm/s may inaccurately calculate the regurgitate volume. An initial velocity of 50 cm/s will be too low and cause aliasing [8].

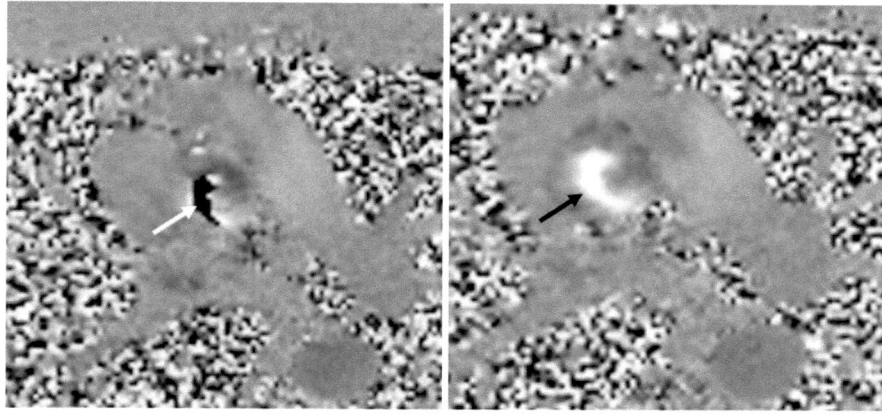

Aliasing (white arrows) at VENC 50cm/s   No aliasing (Black arrow) at 100cm/s

146. A patient is undergoing evaluation of their patent ductus arteriosus, the pulmonary flow is 3.9 L, the aortic flow is 4 L the Qp:Qs is?

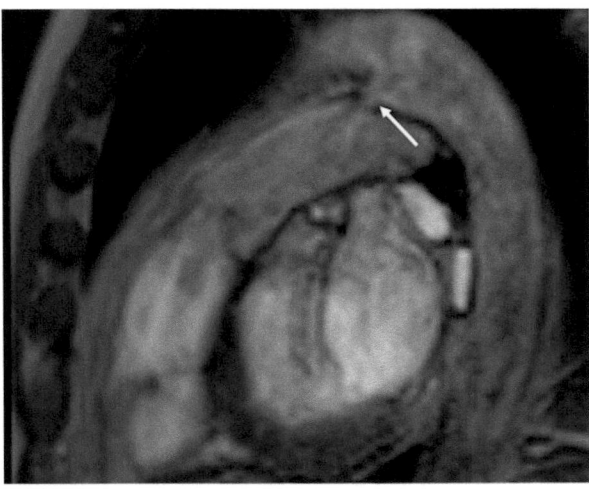

(A) 3.9:4.0
(B) 4.0:3.9
(C) 0.1:1.0
(D) 1.0:0.1

The correct answer is B, 4.0:3.9. When evaluating a patent ductus arteriosus, the aortic flow is the Qp, while the pulmonary flow is the Qs.

147. Which of the following is an indication to calculate a Qp:Qs?

(A) Ventricular septal defect
(B) Atrial septal defect
(C) Patent foramen ovale
(D) Anomalous pulmonary venous return
(E) All the above

The correct answer is E, all of the above. VSD, ASD, PFO, and anomalous pulmonary venous return are all indications to calculate a Qp:Qs to determine if a significant shunt exists.

148. A significant shunt is considered.

(A) Qp:Qs 1.3
(B) Qp:Qs 1
(C) Qp:Qs 1.5
(D) Qp:Qs 0.9

The correct answer is C. A ratio of 1.5 or greater. Shunts of 1.5 or greater lead to left atrial and left ventricular volume overload, leading to elevated pressures and pulmonary hypertension (Rajiah).

149. Qp:Qs is appropriate to be obtained after which of the following?

(A) Percutaneous ASD closure
(B) Surgical VSD closure
(C) Percutaneous PFO closure
(D) A and C
(E) All of the above

The correct answer is E. All of the above are indications to calculate a Qp:Qs to examine if residual shunt remains. While there can be artifact caused by metallic devices and meshes of the closure devices, flow quantification can still be obtained to see if shunt exists and examine the placement of the device.

150. I feel my knowledge of MRI increased since completing this review?

(A) True
(B) False

We hope the correct answer is A. This review is meant to help individuals prepare for the exam. We took countless hours searching and preparing cases and questions. If you feel any topic was not well reviewed or have suggestions, please email mri-guys2022@gmail.com.

References

1. Lotz J, Meier C, Leppert A, Galanski M. Cardiovascular flow measurement with phase-contrast MR imaging: basic facts and implementation. RadioGraphics. 2002;22(3):651–71. https://doi.org/10.1148/radiographics.22.3.g02ma11651.
2. Walker CM, Reddy GP, Mohammed T-LH, Chung JH. Systolic anterior motion of the mitral valve. J Thorac Imaging. 2012;27(4):W87. https://doi.org/10.1097/RTI.0b013e31825412dd.
3. Elster Orbital Foreign Bodies. https://mriquestions.com/orbital-foreign-bodies.html
4. Elster A. Choosing PE & FE directions. https://mriquestions.com/choosing-pefe-direction.html#:~:text=The%20phase%2Dencoding%20direction%20is,in%20the%20phase%2Dencode%20direction. Accessed 10 Jun 2022.
5. Mushabbar S, Mohiaddin R. Magnetic resonance imaging of congenital heart disease. 2012.
6. Srichai MB, Lim RP, Wong S, Lee VS. Cardiovascular applications of phase-contrast MRI. Am J Roentgenol. 2009;192(3):662–75. https://doi.org/10.2214/AJR.07.3744.
7. Chaothawee L. Diagnostic approach to assessment of valvular heart disease using magnetic resonance imaging, part II: a practical approach for native and prosthetic heart valve stenosis. Heart Asia. 2014;4(1):171–5. https://doi.org/10.1136/heartasia-2012-010124.
8. Lee JW, Hur JH, Yang DH, Lee BY, Im DJ, Hong SJ, Kim EY, Park E-A, Jo Y, Kim JJ, Park CH, Yong HS. Guidelines for cardiovascular magnetic resonance imaging from the Korean society of cardiovascular imaging (KOSCI) - Part 2: interpretation of cine, flow, and angiography data. Investig Magn Reson Imaging. 2019;23(4):316. https://doi.org/10.13104/imri.2019.23.4.316.

Index